THE
PICKY
EATING
SOLUTION

THE PICKY EATING SOLUTION

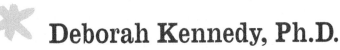

Deborah Kennedy, Ph.D.

Author of *Beat Sugar Addiction Now! for Kids*

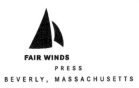

FAIR WINDS
PRESS
BEVERLY, MASSACHUSETTS

© 2013 Fair Winds Press

Text © 2013 Deborah Kennedy, Ph.D.

First published in the USA in 2013 by
Fair Winds Press, a member of
Quarto Publishing Group USA Inc.
100 Cummings Center
Suite 406-L
Beverly, MA 01915-6101
www.fairwindspress.com

ISBN: 978-1-59233-569-5

Digital edition published in 2013
eISBN: 978-1-61058-915-4

Library of Congress Cataloging-in-Publication Data available

Cover and book design by Kathie Alexander
Book layout by Sporto

Printed and bound in U.S.A.

The information in this book is for educational purposes only. It is not intended to replace the advice of a physician or medical practitioner. Please see your health care provider before beginning any new health program.

Dedication

To all the little nuggets out there who struggle with food, this book is for you with love.

This book is dedicated to my children, my friends' children, and the many children I have had the privilege to work with. If it wasn't for watching you and your dance at snack and mealtimes, I wouldn't have been able to look so deeply into the world of feeding. You all continue to inspire and motivate me while you fill my life with joy and love.

A special dedication to my beloved Papa who left this world recently at the age of ninety-three: you continue to inspire me and always will!

Contents

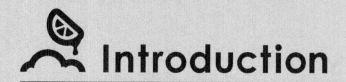# Introduction

Do you want to know whether your children are picky eaters or whether their picky eating will affect their health in a negative way? I suspect that most of you who pick up this book already know the answers to these questions. You know because it is so hard to get your children to eat healthy food that you are at your wit's end. You can't believe that feeding your child a healthy diet has to be so hard, and you hang on to the hope that there must be a better way.

I can honestly say that it doesn't have to be so hard, and there *is* a better way. You will learn exactly what you need to do to turn around your picky eaters—and you do need to turn their eating around if you want them to reach their ultimate potential for health, height, and intelligence.

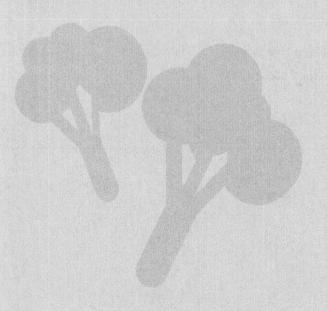

Defining Picky Eating

If you are looking for an official definition of *picky eating,* you will not find it. It is not a term that is considered an official condition or diagnosis; in fact, it is more of a subjective expression. The main reason for this is that picky eating is not considered an official disorder. It does not show up in the medical and mental diagnosis manuals that physicians use to classify patient behaviors under a certain condition or illness. But now that adults are coming forward announcing that they, too, are picky eaters, there is some movement to classify what clinicians call *selective eaters* in adults.

You would think that there would be an official diagnosis for picky eating, seeing that so much attention is focused on the issue. In studies, many researchers just ask parents whether they consider their children to be picky eaters. This makes the term open to interpretation because what may qualify one child to be a picky eater for one parent may not qualify him for another.

Even though there is no universal definitional diagnosis, there are traits that many picky eaters share:

- They eat only a limited variety of foods.

- They will not try new foods readily. Being afraid of trying new foods is referred to as *food neophobia,* and refusing to eat certain foods is called *food aversion.*

Definition or not, this book is for you if you either cannot get your children to eat or it takes an enormous amount of effort for them to eat any of the following foods on a regular basis:

- Three vegetables a day

- Two fruits a day

- Limit of 1 glass (4 to 8 ounces or 120 to 235 ml) of 100 percent juice a day

- At least half their grains as whole grains

- Healthy protein sources such as legumes, fish, and lean meats

- No more than one treat/junk food a day

- No more than one fast food meal once a week

- Sweet drinks such as soda or sports drinks about once a week or less

- Two to three glasses of milk a day (either dairy or an alternative fortified with calcium)

These servings are based on national recommendations or recent scientific findings. For your children to get everything necessary for their growth and long-term health, they need to eat the variety of foods listed here.

But even if your child does not meet one of these conditions, this book is for you. There will be times when feeding your child will be challenging. This book will prepare you to handle the tricks and manipulative techniques children use before they snowball into a picky eating issue.

Are We Programmed to Be Picky Eaters?

We are all born with taste preferences: generally, to avoid bitter-tasting foods and to prefer sweet-tasting ones. This genetic setup helped us survive during a time when we were living off the land as hunters and gatherers and all of our food choices were straight from nature and full of nutrition. The bitter-tasting foods were more likely poisonous while the sweet-tasting ones were usually safe. This survival trait served us very well in the past, but today it is a major contributor to the fight most parents have with getting their children to limit sweets and eat their vegetables.

Not everyone responds to the same degree when it comes to liking sweets and avoiding bitter tastes. Some individuals are supersensitive to bitter tastes while others do not have a problem with them. These supersensitive tasters, or supertasters, are most likely the children who pitch a fit when they are given broccoli while other children do not mind it as much.

I have two sons, and one is very sensitive to bitter tastes while the other is not. Understanding that you may be working with a supertaster can empower you to approach your child in a more compassionate way. If you want to test who in your family is super sensitive to bitter tastes and who isn't, try this experiment: Buy a bottle of tonic water and give everyone a taste. Be prepared for some to spit it out and yell that it tastes disgusting while others do not think that it tastes like much of anything. Next, add some salt to the tonic water and, voilà, those who thought the taste was bitter will now taste sweet (bitter + salty = sweet).

> We are all programmed to go after sweet and avoid bitter tastes, which sets us all up to become picky eaters.

In today's world, this inborn preference for sugary tastes and avoidance of bitter ones creates children who want to eat overly sugary and salty processed foods while refusing to eat their vegetables. In a way, we are all programmed to go after sweet and avoid bitter tastes, which sets us all up to become picky eaters. Once you understand this fact, however, you are well on your way to turning your picky eater around by reinforcing bitter-tasting foods and limiting sweet-tasting ones in your children's diet.

Why is it then that we hear so much about picky eating as if it is a condition that our children suffer from and that we need to treat? I believe it is because standard feeding recommendations do not work in our current food environment. Instead of focusing on our children's food environment, we have targeted our children, as if something is wrong with them when, in fact, they are doing what they are programmed to do. A 2008 study in the *International Journal of Eating Disorders* does not support the concept that picky eating is associated with disordered eating but rather with a range of behavioral problems. It is wise for us to concentrate on the behavioral issues at hand instead of the terminology.

It's Not Just About How You Feed Them

If you have a picky eater in your home, you may feel that you have failed in some way, especially if feeding your child a healthy diet has become impossible in your home. You have *not* failed. Most parents I see have tried everything to get their children to eat healthfully. The trouble with doing "everything" is that it is based on an old theory of feeding kids that has reached its limit of usefulness. It is time for a new way, a way of feeding children in a land full of junk food where children need to use their cognition instead of relying solely on their taste buds. To understand this issue of picky eating better, consider these three contributors to the eating equation:

- **Your child's likes and dislikes.** This is what I see driving the quality of our children's diets today. If you ask them to select what they want to eat without encouraging them to select the healthy options available, most children choose only the super-yummy, heavily processed options.

- **Your child's food environment.** Picky eating hasn't changed over the years, but our children's food environment has transformed drastically. Children today have no concept of where food comes from, so to them anything can look like food, including glow-in-the-dark candy.

- **Your parenting feeding style.** The way we interact with our children around food influences if and how they will eat. Most of us were advised to let our children decide what they will and will not eat, which will most likely not work when feeding picky eaters. In the next chapter, you will learn what parenting style works the best and what your feeding style is.

Much of the literature on picky eating has focused on one part of the equation: how parents are supposed to manipulate their child's eating habits so they eat healthfully. This book looks at all elements of the eating equation together and creates a plan for you to deal with your child's individual eating style and how best to work with your child in his or her current food environment—one that is so full of junk food at every turn that our children have a one in two (for Hispanic and African-American children) or one in three chance of getting diabetes in their lifetime and a one in three chance of becoming overweight.

Let's get rid of the term *picky eating* and call it what it truly is: deficient eating. A deficient eater is one whose pickiness is serious enough to potentially affect his or her health. Some children who are labeled picky eaters may not be consuming adequate calories while others are getting a surplus of calories, and still others may be getting adequate calories, but are consuming a low or deficient amount of the micronutrients they need to reach their potential and live a healthy life.

Even though we are all born preferring sweets and avoiding bitter tastes, why is it that some children grow up to eat a healthy diet while others do not? I suspect it has a lot to do with their parents' feeding style and children's unique eating personalities.

Is It Picky Eating or a Sensory Issue?

It is important to take a brief moment to explain tactile dysfunction and a related disorder called sensory food aversion (SFA). SFA is different from what many of us call picky eating, although being a picky eater is one symptom of it. SFA affects a small number of children. These children have difficulty with food as do picky eaters, but they also have difficulty integrating different senses in their life. Children with SFA have a very strong aversion to a food's taste, texture, smell, or temperature but have other sensory difficulties in general as well.

They may have an issue with touch (tactile dysfunction), loud sounds, bright lights, and strong smells, for example. Children who have an aversion to touch, especially light touch, have what is called tactile defensiveness. Many of these children have a hard time with the texture and feel of food in their mouths.

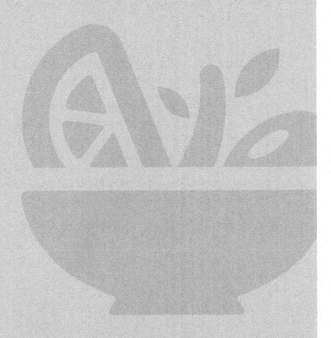

Are you stressing yourself using cookie cutters
to make fun sandwich shapes or feel like
you need an art class to turn veggies
into cute little animal sculptures?
Stop it now!

Such sensory defensiveness is not common, but answer the following questions to get a sense of whether a sensory dysfunction may be affecting your child's eating habits:

- Did your child have trouble with breast-feeding or bottle-feeding?

- Did your child's picky eating begin after he was introduced to a new food that he really didn't like?

- Has your child gagged or vomited when eating a new food?

- When stage 3 food (pureed food with small bites added in) was introduced to your baby, did she have a strong negative reaction to it and resist eating it?

- In your opinion, or on the diagnosis of a professional, would your child be deficient in nutrients if he did not take a nutritional supplement?

- Did your child develop oral motor and expressive speech delays between birth and age three?

- Does your child get anxious when her hands are messy, teeth are brushed, or shirt label touches her neck? Does your child get anxious when she walks on sand or grass or wears certain fabrics?

- Is your child anxious during mealtime? Does he avoid social situations where food is involved?

If you answered yes to many of the questions above, it is probably wise to follow up with your child's pediatrician to rule out sensory dysfunction or SFA. You can also go to the website of Zero to Three, a national nonprofit, at http://main.zerotothree.org/site/DocServer/29-3_Chatoorv.pdf for a great description of SFA for parents of children up to three years of age. Also, *Raising a Sensory Smart Child* by Lindsey Biel and Nancy Peske is a helpful book on sensory issues in children.

If your child is affected by SFA, you can still use the advice in this book while you work with your pediatrician or occupational therapist.

Food Myth Buster

You have come to the right place if you picked up this book because you have had it with trying to get your children to eat healthy foods, are tired of turning their sandwiches into smiley faces so they will eat them, or are angry at being told that you need to step back and wait for your children to choose to eat their broccoli. Let me start by busting some myths and old-fashioned theories for you:

- **Eating should center on being FUN!** What have we done to ourselves? To start with, we listened to commercials and advice from professionals telling us that if we make eating fun, our kids will eat healthfully. We are brainwashed into believing that to be a good parent we need to put a smile on our kids' faces with the food we put in front of them. You have seen those commercials with kids dancing down the stairs for cinnamon buns or toaster cakes for breakfast. You most likely have swallowed the guilt and think that if your children are not enjoying their meal, then you have failed them. Are you stressing yourself using cookie cutters to make fun sandwich shapes or feel like you need an art class to turn their veggies into cute little animal sculptures? Stop it now! There is a place for fun, but it certainly is not a priority when feeding your child.

- **My child will grow out of picky eating.** I have met and worked with many parents who have been told by their pediatrician to let their child be when it comes to eating healthy food, which usually means vegetables. They are told that their child will, in the future, eat what they are currently refusing. Hogwash! You will learn from this book why this belief goes against science. Children will learn to like the healthy stuff because you have taught them to, plain and simple. In fact, the new term you learned about earlier—selective eating—is being promoted as a mental health condition because adults are admitting that they are picky eaters, too.

- **My child will get all the nutrients he needs if I leave him alone and don't bother him about how he eats.** If I were writing this book in the early 1900s, then you would be right, but not today. A lot has changed since then, especially when it comes to the type of foods and beverages we consume on a daily basis. Today the majority of our child's food choices are processed foods that are heavily marketed to youth while being hyperpalatable. This fancy word just means that food scientists have spent decades trying to figure out how to make certain foods so super-tasty that we can't stop eating them. Children will choose super-yummy food over the healthy stuff almost every time, so leaving them alone is not a good idea if you regularly serve processed or premade food that is high in sugar or salt.

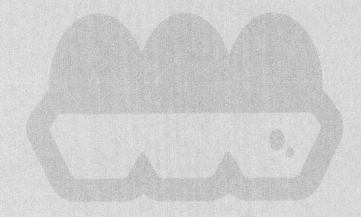

- **Interacting with my children at the dinner table to encourage healthful eating will have negative consequences later in their life.** This antiquated theory was proposed in the 1980s when a small amount of research suggested that children, mostly girls, who had authoritarian parents were at an increased risk of developing an eating disorder later in life.

  There may certainly have been some truth to that, but what this finding has led to thirty-plus years later is the mantra heard at most pediatricians' and dieticians' offices: *You decide the what and where and your child decides the if and how much.* This advice may seem benign, but it has led to one, if not two, generations of parents who have backed off when it comes to teaching their child what foods they need to eat to be healthy. You will learn the right and wrong way to interact with your child at the dinner table, but that doesn't mean you shouldn't teach them what's healthy to eat.

- **My child is healthy as long as he or she is growing.** There is much more to good health then making sure your child's growth is steady. As a nutritionist, one measure—among many others—that I rely on when assessing a child's nutritional health is his growth curve. In practice, as long as your child is staying on that curve, even if he is at the low end, all is considered to be fine in traditional practices. Unless your child has other symptoms, pediatricians and nutritionists usually do not dig any further.

  If your child falls off the curve, then the professionals look deeper. For example, if your child is always at the 25th percentile and suddenly dips to the 15th or jumps to the 40th percentile, there would be a follow-up to determine why that occurred. Nutritionists would look at a child's daily intake of food to determine whether she is getting enough of the healthy building blocks that she needs.

  In my training to become a nutritionist, I was taught about two kinds of malnutrition: one has to do with protein deficiency and the other with total calorie deficiency. When you see pictures of children starving in Africa or India, you are struck by these haunting images of children with swollen bellies (protein deficiency) or some who are so thin you can see their skeleton (total calorie malnutrition). As a society, we have a lot of compassion for people suffering from hunger, and rightly so.

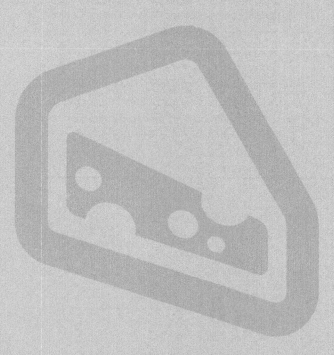

Children come into this world with their own unique personalities, and they do not turn them off when they sit down to eat.

In my training, however, I was not taught about another form of malnutrition that is prevalent today: the one where children get enough calories (even too many) and are overweight, but are still deficient in the micronutrients that they need to live a healthy life. As a society, we have less compassion for individuals suffering from this form of malnutrition because some consider the increased weight a sign of indulgence or gluttony. We need to look beyond that to see that many of our children are actually suffering from nutritional deficiencies.

Measuring growth does nothing to identify whether your child's immune system, intellectual capabilities, and bone health are at their best. A lot can happen inside their body even though they appear healthy on the outside. Monitoring growth is really about making sure enough calories are getting in, but that is only the tip of the iceberg.

I am here to tell you that even though your children are growing, they may not be setting their bodies up to reach their maximum potential—in more ways than one. What your children eat at a very young age sets the foundation for their health later in life. A strong foundation includes fruits and vegetables, healthy fats, protein sources, and whole grains. If your children refuse to eat any of the above, then they are risking not meeting their potential and endangering their health later on, too.

- **Turning around a picky eater takes a lot of hard work.** If you follow the current advice, then yes, turning around a picky eater is hard. The reason for this is that no one has helped you to identify what your child's eating personality is. You wouldn't try to teach a shy child to make new friends in the same way that you would teach an outgoing child. Children come into this world with their own unique personalities, and they do not turn them off when they sit down to eat.

In this book, you will learn how to interact with your child when it comes to food and feeding. Armed with the knowledge of your child's eating personality, plus techniques you can use to help him or her specifically interact with food, will significantly reduce the strife and effort needed to turn around your picky eater.

Labeling a child a picky eater does little to help parents work with their child at the dinner table. *Picky eater* is really a catchall phrase that has become an excuse for both pediatricians and parents to allow unhealthy eating to go on for far too long. The fact is that the majority of children are picky eaters, and the rest have bouts of picky eating here and there. Read on for instructions to help your children thrive in the current food environment. First, though, learn why it is so important that you turn your child's unhealthy eating habits around.

The Life of Bryan

You have probably heard some of the alarming health statistics that this generation of children faces today. Rather than bombard you with more statistics, let's look at the story of Bryan, my three-year old, and project what is in store for him if I follow the current advice and feed him a typical American diet (neither of which I do).

If I were writing this book just a decade ago, I would have probably started this section when I first introduced him to solid food. But in the past ten years there have been a lot of advances in understanding the relationship between influences in the womb and later eating preferences.

So let's begin at the beginning. Bryan is conceived and his genetic footprint is formed. The way that his genes will be expressed will depend on not just what is written in his genes but also by his environment. What this means is that what I choose to eat while pregnant with him will affect the way his genes are expressed. His taste preferences are beginning to form while growing inside of me. How wild is that? If I eat more vegetables, he will be more likely to enjoy vegetables when he is introduced to them.

On the other hand, if I am following the standard American diet (SAD) while pregnant, Bryan is being exposed to unhealthy trans and saturated fats, with limited essential fatty acids. This fat profile is already starting to affect his IQ potential. He will get bathed in sugar from all the processed food and beverages that I am consuming. He won't be exposed to the taste of vegetables because I am not eating them. This will set him up to have a harder time with vegetables, and he will be more likely to overeat and crave junk food.

It is now the day of his birth, and he is immediately placed on my belly to bond. This early connection with me, his mother, is essential. Think about it: He was all warm and cozy inside the womb, and with birth, he bursts forth into a room full of bright lights, activity, and sound. He begins to learn that a physical connection is soothing and that mom and dad are there to protect him. I put him to my breast to see if he wants to suckle and—bam!—the food and self-soothing connection begins. I begin my nine- to twelve-month intimate bond with him by breast-feeding, which will provide all the nutrients he needs. If I provide the comfort, connection, and nourishment from not just a physical perspective but an emotional one as well and continue to feed his needs both physically and emotionally as he grows, he may not be as tempted to choose food later on to soothe himself.

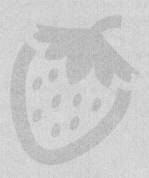

When I introduce vegetables, if [Bryan] makes a face I will stop right away if I don't understand that just a new taste will cause this facial expression.

Instead of that, though, he will most likely be whisked away immediately after birth to be cleaned up, measured, and stuck with needles. He will come back so fussy that I will have a hard time beginning to breast-feed. If no one has taught me, I may struggle and feel like a failure when breast-feeding does not come easily, which it rarely does. If I don't know that breast-feeding may be quite painful in the beginning, I may give up reluctantly (or be secretly pleased) and turn to bottle-feeding. Bryan will be given a formula that has as its number one ingredient high-fructose corn syrup. All this sugar will set him up to want more and more of it.

Fast-forward through the first six months and the bottle versus breast milk conflict: Breast milk is healthier but necessity sometimes warrants moms to bottle-feed. Breast milk actually provides a better nutrient profile than bottled milk to a growing baby. It also supplies agents to help Bryan's intestinal tract go from one where in utero he was receiving all his nutrients through the umbilical cord to one where he now needs to use his intestinal tract to absorb nutrients.

There are factors in my breast milk to help digest his food, protect him from an immune perspective, and help his intestines mature. Introducing other foods before his intestines have matured could potentially lead to an increased incidence of food allergies, although science is still mixed on that issue. Having an older child with severe food allergies makes me more cautious in introducing solid food to Bryan at a young age, so I wait a little longer to do so.

To determine when it is time to offer Bryan table food, I will wait for him to give me cues that he is ready: He will reach for my food, mimic my chewing, and give me a strong message through his body language that he wants to try real food. I will start by offering him some whole grain cereal and then advance to vegetables, saving the sweet fruits for later. Bryan will gobble up the jarred and pureed fruits and vegetables, and he will eat what I offer to him.

If I listen to the standard advice from pediatricians, though, I will introduce food when Bryan is six months old. I most likely will start with processed grain and then advance to fruits. If I want my baby to sleep through the night, I may stick cereal into his bottle if I don't know any better because a friend suggested it. Or I will be so excited about feeding him new food that I will begin feeding him baby food as early as three months—at a time when his intestines are not developed enough to handle it. My pediatrician may or may not discourage that. When I introduce vegetables, he may or may not like them, but if he makes a face I will stop right away if I don't understand that just a new taste will cause this facial expression. He will gobble up most of his pureed fruits and grains until I introduce him to processed food.

The track that I take in the first six months of Bryan's life will predispose him to crave sweeter and sweeter food or not; to set up his intestinal tract to be healthy so he does not develop allergies or sensitivities to food later in his life or cause damage to his gut so that he will be sensitive to lots of foods; and I, as a parent, will either work with his cues or go against them. Either way, I have a child who eats pretty well at six months. Most six- to twelve-month-olds I see and work with are eating a pretty healthy diet of jarred fruits and vegetables or homemade baby food. Most babies will continue to eat the whole foods they are offered: ground-up protein, cereal, and fruits and vegetables. It isn't until babies are introduced to processed foods that we begin to see the struggles with eating. I am not talking about pureed food but food that has additives, sweeteners, and salt: soda, juice, cookies, salty crackers made with processed white flour, pudding, and much more.

The first 6 months of Bryan's life is as easy as it gets in terms of feeding him, because he is relying mostly on breast milk and pureed wholesome fruits or vegetables. Once children taste "the other side"—the artificially high sweet, salty, and savory tastes of foods and beverages that have added chemicals, flavors, sugar, and salt—they do not want to go back. If you understand that whole food can never compete tastewise with processed food, then you are armed with the single most important piece of information that you need to bring up a healthy eater.

If I didn't encourage Bryan to eat the healthy stuff first before he could have the treats, or didn't continue to offer vegetables until he developed a taste for them, or didn't refuse to make another dinner if he didn't like the one I cooked for him, then he would be running the show like most children do today. He would be led by his taste buds, and before you knew it, he would be getting most of his calories from desserts followed by pizza and then soda and energy and sports drinks. This statistic, from the Dietary Guidelines for Americans 2010, is the result of parents not setting rules and consequences at the dinner table.

As a nutritionist and a mother, I was prepared to fight the fight with Bryan each and every day. What I mean is that I knew if I left it up to him, he would drink his milk and eat lots of dessert but choose not to eat his dinner. I saw early on that he was a *Drinker* and a *Junk Food Junkie* (see chapter 6 to read about all five eating personalities). He would rather drink his calories than eat them. He was always off and running and wanted to play and had trouble sitting down at meal times. He was also my son who was not satisfied with one cookie but wanted three or four, whereas my older son was happy and content with one or two cookies. Knowing which eating personalities I was working with helped me to set rules and consequences that worked specifically for Bryan. He understood at twelve months old that to get milk he first had to eat a few bites of dinner. The technique of "first this, then that" worked well for him and still does. *First eat dinner, then you can have dessert* is a nightly ritual at my dinner table. It is not a struggle but a matter-of-fact conversation that I have with him.

If you understand that whole food can never compete tastewise with processed food, then you are armed with the single most important piece of information that you need to bring up a healthy eater.

If I didn't understand anything about eating personalities and followed the current guidelines, I would have put Bryan's food and milk in front of him at dinnertime and watched as he downed his milk, asked for more, and then ate maybe one or two bites of dinner before announcing that he was full. I would take him at his word and excuse him from the table only to have him come up to me ten minutes later asking for dessert. I would give him ice cream and if he were still hungry, off I would trek on the after-dinner snacking trail where he would eat probably four hundred calories in chips, cookies, gummy fruit, and many others of his favorite treats.

This would go on for years and I would watch as he ate little to no vegetables and preferred only the standard kid fare of mac 'n' cheese, pizza, hot dogs, and chicken nuggets and drank lots of sugar-sweetened beverages. He would go from preferring his bottle when he was a toddler to chocolate milk, then sports drinks and flavored water followed by soda and energy drinks as he got older. At the age of seven or eight he would most likely be consuming his weight in sugar every year.

In the back of my mind I would think that this could not be healthy for him, but every time I bring it up to the pediatrician she would say not to worry, that Bryan is growing well, he isn't overweight, and he is healthy. I would occasionally read something in the press that would say yet again how vegetables were really important, and I would try to get Bryan to eat them. I would serve broccoli with dip or add melted cheese to it. I may even go so far as to make his vegetables into fun little critter shapes only to have him maybe take a bite or two. Because I am a busy working parent, I give up after a short while because I really don't have the time to keep doing this—and it doesn't seem to be that effective anyway. As long as Bryan is happy and not screaming at the table, then my job is done. Or is it?

I think we can all say with confidence
that the current guidance is not working and
children are suffering needlessly from the dire
consequences of eating a diet of too much
junk and not enough healthy food.

This eating habit, a diet high in sugar and solid fats and low in fruits, vegetables, and whole grains, will lead to Bryan having a real risk of becoming overweight or obese and developing many health risks. Here is just a sampling: He will be at an increased risk for developing asthma, sleep apnea, liver and gallbladder disease, and bone and joint problems. He will have a hard time exercising because he will be out of breath, and socially he will have a rough time. He may turn to abusing drugs or alcohol, becoming bulimic or anorexic, plus he will probably be depressed. He could start to put down plaque, which leads to heart disease, when he is in elementary school, and he may need to take heart medication as an adolescent to prevent a heart attack when he is a teenager or a young adult.

Even if he doesn't become overweight, loading his system with this much sugar, solid fat, and artificial chemicals will still stress his pancreas, which will most likely lead to diabetes. Eating all these chemicals and junk food will most likely cause him to be hyperactive, and he will need medication to settle down.

His immune system will not be at its best because he is not receiving the optimal levels of micronutrients. His bowel health will probably be compromised because he is getting so little fiber. Most likely he will become constipated, which will mean that the toxins in his stool will have more time to cause damage to the intestines, which can lead to an increased risk of colon cancer if it continues over a prolonged period of time. His gut may be inflamed as well, and this inflammation may spread to the rest of his body where it can damage his joints over the years. The solid fats and trans fat that he is consuming in large amounts from the processed food will increase his risk for heart disease. So you see, even if Bryan doesn't become overweight by eating a diet high in junk food, his body is still being affected in a multitude of negative, unhealthy ways.

If you hear some of your child's eating history in this fictitious but oh-so-true story of Bryan, do not despair. This book is dedicated to you, the mom or dad who cares so much for your child that you are willing to do anything to help your child reach his or her potential and be as healthy as can be.

I think we can all say with confidence that the current guidance is not working and children are suffering needlessly from the dire consequences of eating a diet of too much junk and not enough healthy food. If we continue to put junk in our children's bodies and medicate them from the harm that this type of food produces, we are setting them up for a life filled with many health conditions: heart disease, certain cancers, diabetes, and other negative health consequences, including not living as long as their parents. This is exactly what the science is showing.

But here is the good news: Most, if not all, of this can be turned around by the choices we make for our children every day. Each time our children choose an apple over a gummy fruit bar or low-fat milk over chocolate milk, they are moving on a path toward health and wellness.

Let's begin in section 1 by first empowering you to take back your control over what your child eats. You will determine your unique feeding style and learn which feeding behaviors are effective. I will show you the rules and consequences that need to be in place to teach your children how to live a healthy life as well as train their taste buds to like the healthy stuff. You will also learn a six-step process for setting the stage at mealtime, which encourages healthy eating and minimizes chaos. In section 2, you will learn how to identify your child's unique eating personality and work with his or her natural tendencies in creating a healthy eater. Let's begin!

Tools for Parents to Turn Their
Picky Eater Around

CHAPTER 1

Empowering Parents at Mealtime

Does dinnertime fill you with dread and maybe a touch of fear? Are you so exhausted after a long day that you just don't have it in you to fight the battle of getting your kids to eat a healthy meal? Perhaps you have already given up so you pick up some fast food or take-home from the grocery store because you know they won't fight you on this. Who can blame you? Not me.

We all want our kids to be happy and healthy, and if fast-food makes them happy and reduces your stress at dinner, what's the harm? Lots! That is why I wrote this book: to convince you that if your children are not eating the recommended amount of healthy food, then their health will suffer regardless of whether they have weight issues or are considered picky eaters.

Blame never leads to anything constructive, so be assured that there will be none of that here—and, in reality, there is no one to blame. You, along with most parents, have been disempowered by the current feeding recommendation that focuses on letting the child decide what to eat. It is based on an antiquated theory that just doesn't work anymore because we live in a world full of processed food that is cheap, easy to find, and very tasty. The goal of this book is to give you your power back when it comes to feeding your children and provide you with tools that work for your individual eater.

A Real-World Example

At my son's fourth birthday party, I was disheartened and amused at the same time over what I saw happening at the picnic table. I gave a lot of thought to what food I would serve to a group of four-year-olds, knowing that some would probably be picky. In fact, I counted on it. I decided on pinwheels: turkey with mayo wrapped up in a tortilla with a cucumber in the middle. I knew that adding the cucumber was taking a chance and even experienced a bit of anxiety over it. Can you believe that I was nervous over what the response from the little partygoers would be?

As expected, I saw a couple of children pick the cucumber out of the wrap before they would eat their sandwich, but others played out a scene that I would describe as comedy if the consequences of unhealthy eating weren't so tragic. One mother pleaded with her daughter to take another bite after she separated the meat from the wrap, broke the food up into microscopic pieces, and fed it to her daughter like she was a baby bird.

Another mom was faced with screams of "No!" and a shake of the head and kicking when she asked her son to eat the wrap; she gave up quickly, embarrassed. That mom told me that the night before, her son didn't want to eat the chicken they had ordered at a restaurant, so after it was served and he took two bites, out it came all over the table. I respected her valiant effort and was saddened by how ineffective her efforts were despite trying so hard. There was also another child who wouldn't eat no matter how much her mom begged.

It is time for you to start running the show again. It can be done, and you don't have to be militant or angry to do it.

Of the seven partygoers, two wouldn't eat at all, three were very picky, and two were great eaters. I ask you, who was in charge here? The kids, that is for sure! I felt and saw the power dynamic clear as day: The parent was intimidated and the child was the boss.

The scene at my son's party encapsulates what is happening at most every dinner table across this country on most nights of the week. Parents cower in fear and confusion, and my heart goes out to each and every one of you. I know that you are just following the national recommendation to back off and let your child decide what he or she wants to eat. I am here to tell you that this method is not working—which is probably a relief to many of you because, in your heart of hearts, you know it isn't working either.

If any of these statements describes you, there is help:

- I cross my fingers when I put dinner on the table and hope that my child will eat it.

- I will make another meal if my child doesn't like what I served at mealtime.

- I miss eating regular food because all I serve is kid fare: nuggets, mac 'n' cheese, and hot dogs.

- I am so tired at the end of the long day that I will let my child eat dessert and after-dinner snacks even if he didn't eat enough of his dinner.

- I get embarrassed when we go out to a restaurant or a friend's house because I know my son will pitch a fit if I say no to his request for a third juice box.

- I serve my child only foods that I know she likes.

- I have given up on vegetables because I know my child will not eat them no matter what I do.

- Dinnertime is okay unless one of my children yells "Yuck!" and then the rest of my children will not eat their dinner either.

It is time for you to start running the show again. It can be done, and you don't have to be militant or angry to do it. At that same party, I watched as a three-year old asked his mom whether he could have some juice. I could tell immediately that his mom was in charge and if she said no, then he would move on to something else. Contrast his reaction to that of most children at birthday parties. They ask, but "yes" is the only answer they want. Their mom knows it, their dad knows it, and most important, the children know it, too!

How to Introduce Variety into Your Child's Diet

It takes children ten to fifteen tries to "like" a new food. For children on the autism spectrum, it can take many more attempts—upwards of fifty or one hundred. Many of us believe that if we give our children a new food and they spit it out, it means they were born not liking it. That is an obvious and valid conclusion—if you didn't know that children need to *learn* to like new foods.

Most babies will make a face when presented with a new taste; that is just because they have never tried that food before. It doesn't mean you should stop giving it to them. With a toddler or young child, start by giving him one bite of a new food and slowly increase his exposure to the new food over time, asking for two bites the next time, and so on, until he becomes accustomed to the taste.

As a parent, you will know which foods you can encourage and which foods are true "yucky" foods. On a scale of 0 to 5, with 5 representing "I love it" and 1 meaning "I can't stand it and may just throw up," I never want you to encourage your child to eat foods that score a 0 to 1; those are the foods that are super-yucky to children—so bad, in fact, they just might gag or vomit when asked to eat it. You will find, however, that many foods lie in the 2 to 4 range. These are foods your child may not prefer and say they don't like, but if encouraged, they will learn to like them after repeated exposure. You will learn more about how to do this in chapter 3, when the one-bite rule is discussed.

Generally speaking, not many foods fall at either the 0 or 5 extreme; most foods lie in the middle of the scale. It is perfectly acceptable and even wise to offer those foods in the middle of the scale—it is the only way you will introduce variety into your children's diet. When your child says "Yuck!" about foods that are in the 0 to 4 range and you take her at face value, you are left serving your child only the foods that she will gobble down without a fight. That would be great if the foods that most children loved were more nutritional—not processed, usually beige in color, with added salt and sugar, and little-to-no fiber in sight. We know these foods, as they are on almost all children's menus at restaurants and in school cafeterias.

A History Lesson

Early research on parents' practices surrounding their children's eating habits looked at their general parenting framework—whether they were authoritarian or indulgent, for example—and how that affected their children's diet. This was a good place to start, but there is a big problem with generalizing a parenting style across all situations because most parents know that their parenting style depends on the specific circumstance. You may be strict with your child about homework, for example, but when it comes to going to bed you are permissive. Your style often depends on what you want your children to do, and you most likely approach each of these areas differently. Also, you may have a child with whom you need to intervene when it comes to homework, but another child who needs little to no oversight in that area.

The same holds true with eating. It is not accurate to predict how a general parenting style will affect a child's eating habits, which is probably why results are all over the place about a specific parenting style and its effectiveness in establishing healthy eating practices. A more accurate question is "How does my feeding style influence my specific child?" Research has not answered that question yet.

Early research in the 1980s suggested that having an authoritarian parent had an influence on children, specifically girls, developing eating disorders later in life. This was followed by a series of books that promoted "Parents are responsible for the what, when, and where of feeding; children are responsible for the how much and whether of feeding." Many, many parents were helped with this advice. Fast-forward thirty years, and, as a consequence of this recommendation, many parents today have backed off and inadvertently given their children free reign at the table and in the grocery store.

As a child of a very militant father, I am personally glad that someone promoted not forcing children to eat. My grandparents lived through the Great Depression, and "making children eat" was a survival behavior. My dad was born during this time when food was scarce; in turn, he passed along the feeding behavior he was exposed to: "Eat what is served, no exceptions." My four brothers and sisters and I had to eat everything that was served. We were screamed at and threatened if we did not. You may think this behavior was mean—and I won't say it was not—but my father was doing what he was taught to do and what he saw everyone else doing.

I think the pendulum has swung in the opposite direction a bit too far: There is too much leniency at the dinner table.

Aren't most parents today doing what they are taught and what they see everyone else doing, even if it doesn't feel right? I think the pendulum has swung in the opposite direction a bit too far: There is too much leniency at the dinner table. Parents needed to change the clean-your-plate rule when it was determined that this was an unhealthy feeding practice that was no longer needed because they weren't living during an economic depression. I believe we are at another turning point now, a time when our current food environment warrants a new feeding practice that helps parents promote healthy eating in the overly processed world.

We cannot put our children in control at a time when they have access to junk food wherever they turn. Sixteen percent of their calories come from added sugar, and processed food is addictive. It is time for those who know best—parents—to take the power back. In this book, you will be encouraged to get involved in your children's food lives. You will discover that taste is learned, some food is addictive, and how best to establish healthy eating patterns. You will be instructed to set rules and consequences and encourage your children on a daily basis. This chapter describes why parents' power needs to be returned: Your children's lives are at stake!

Now that you have an idea of how we got here—to a place where our kids are running the show and to a place where many are confused and maybe have even given up at mealtime—it's time to learn how to get out of here. The direction of where to go from here will become clearer once you learn more about your feeding style and determine which feeding practices are effective with your children.

The Hard Facts on Parental Feeding Styles

I always like to explain the bottom-line of scientific findings to make them easier to understand. Research into different parental feeding styles and the effects of these styles on children's eating behaviors, however, are all over the place, so it's difficult to draw a conclusion based on the current findings. For example, when you look at the effects of restricting unhealthy food, some studies find that it leads to children eating more of the forbidden food and having a higher body mass index, whereas others find it effective in limiting unhealthy food intake.

Figuring out how to feed your children doesn't have to be complicated.

Parents who promote and stimulate healthy eating have been shown to have a favorable outcome in certain studies and an unfavorable outcome in others. I believe, and studies suggest, that these different findings may be the result of a one-size-does-not-fit-all—that is, one parenting approach does not fit all children. How could it?

There are two personalities at work in a feeding dyad: the parent's and the child's. We all know that what might work for strong-willed children most likely will not work for easygoing children. For example, restricting unhealthy food for a strong-willed child may backfire but for an easygoing child it may be successful. In fact, a 2011 Netherlands study looking at family feeding practices showed that if a child was labeled "picky," he or she tended to react negatively to restriction of unhealthy food but positively to monitoring and stimulating healthy food intake. The study authors concluded, "The associations between several of the parenting practices and child behavior were found to depend on child characteristics, which calls for parenting that is tailored to each individual child." That is what this book is all about!

Figuring out how to feed your children doesn't have to be complicated. In a nutshell, you know which practices work for getting your children to do what you want them to do, like brushing their teeth, cleaning up their room, and sharing their toys. I will help you figure out how to use this information to get them to eat healthfully. In the following text, you will discover your feeding style, and in section 2, you will determine which eating personality—the Easygoing Eater, the Anxious Eater, the Strong-Willed Eater, the Distracted Eater, and the Taster—best fits your child. This information will be essential for you to learn how to work with your child at the table. In addition, there are a number of characters that fall under the five eating personalities; enjoy finding your child in one or more of these (such as the Drinker, the Short Order Diner, Mr./Miss Bland, or the Gobbler).

What Is Your Feeding Style?

A lot of factors went into and continue to create your distinct feeding style, some of which you can control and others that you cannot. They include the following:

- **Ethnicity:** Each ethnic group has unique ways of feeding that are passed among members of its community. Take a look at your heritage and determine if the feeding practices help or hinder your efforts.

- **How you were fed as a child:** Your family history has a major influence on how you feed your child. The way your parents interacted with you around food strongly affects your feeding style. You may use your parents' practices, or if you had a negative experience with those practices, you may have made a conscious choice to not repeat your parents' feeding style. In either case, the way you were brought up at the table influences your current feeding style.

- **Your personality:** Your personality plays a major role in how you approach your child at the table. Whether you are laid back or intense will determine how you interact with your child. Depending on your child's personality, your own personality may connect with her or rub her the wrong way.

- **You or your child's current weight:** Research suggests that you will approach feeding your child differently if you or he is overweight. Parents who are concerned that their child is over- or underweight exercise more control over what their child eats than those parents who have no concerns for their child's health. If you are overweight, that also adds another layer of influence. Research demonstrates that moms who are obese feed their children more when their children are emotionally distressed. They use food as a reward, and they encourage their child to eat more than moms who are not obese.

- **Concerns with your child's health:** If you are worried about your child's health, you most likely will monitor her intake more than if she had no health issues.

The type of parenting that elicits the most positive outcomes for children, as a whole, is the authoritative parenting style.

The more controllable factors that go into creating your feeding style—such as your stress level, time crunches, money issues, pets, and siblings—will be discussed in chapter 4. You will learn how to overcome or deal with your current environment to best create a healthy eater.

Four Feeding Styles

There is a well-subscribed-to and accepted theory of parenting styles developed initially by Diana Baumrind, Ph.D., a clinical and developmental psychologist. She observed preschool children and discovered three distinct parenting styles, which were later expanded by others to include a fourth. The four parenting style categories are authoritarian, authoritative, indulgent, and uninvolved. The type of parenting that elicits the most positive outcomes for children, as a whole, is the authoritative parenting style. Studies show that children who have this type of parent are happier, successful, and capable.

Following is a description of these parenting styles, focusing particularly on how each pertains to eating. You will discover which style you use most often, but remember that your feeding style will be situation-specific and influenced by the factors covered earlier, plus your child's age and current environment. Also, your spouse may or may not have the same parenting style as you do.

The goal of this chapter is for you to learn about the four feeding styles and discover which one you use most often with each of your children. For example, you may be indulgent when it comes to how you interact with your children in a restaurant, but authoritative when eating meals at home.

Mr./Mrs. Strict: The Authoritarian Parent at the Table

Authoritarian parents are big on control and overriding a child's preference. They are demanding of their children and unresponsive to their demands. The parent's agenda is the only one that matters. The authoritarian parent is president of the clean-your-plate club.

Whether a child wants or doesn't want a certain food is of no concern to authoritarians. They sometimes use physical force, yelling, and screaming to get their child to eat and can be pretty scary at times. This type of behavior causes a lot of anxiety at the table and could be related to the increases seen in studies of eating disorders in female college students in the 1980s and 1990s.

Authoritarian parents can also be inconsistent, making some meals a battle while leaving others alone. Sometimes they will let transgressions go and other times they don't. Either way, children are always expecting the hammer to fall when they have an authoritarian parent at the table.

As I said earlier, this was my father's parenting style when it came to eating at the dinner table. My brothers and sisters and I could not leave the table until everything was eaten. I still to this day cringe when I even hear someone mention creamed corn. (I am slightly gagging even as I write this!) My dad made me sit for hours until I ate the creamed corn, by then cold, left on my plate.

If you find that this feeding style resonates with how you currently feed your child, do not be upset with yourself. This feeding style is old school and was most likely developed during the Depression and at other times in our history when food was scarce, survival was at stake, and parents needed their children to eat to live. In this environment, the authoritarian style of feeding was necessary and would be again if food was so scarce that our children's survival was at stake.

If you can't imagine easing up on the reins because you truly believe you need force to get your children to eat, read on. The next part of this chapter describes how you can still be authoritative without being forceful and how to take your children's desires and needs into account without giving up your control.

The authoritarian feeding style is too strict for most children. It is perfectly acceptable and even encouraged to set rules and consequences at the table, but these must be enforced with the children's needs in mind to be most effective.

The Teacher/Coach: The Authoritative Parent at the Table

Authoritative parents do a great balancing act between being authoritarian and permissive. They have a high degree of control, but they are also very responsive to their children. Authoritative parents listen and read their children's cues at the table. Their children's desires are important, and so is the parent's need to get them to eat a healthy diet. These parents use nurturing, reasoning, and structure to encourage children to eat. If authoritative parents want their children to clean their plate, they encourage them to do so, tell them why it is important, and make sure they give them an appropriate portion of food. Recent research is most supportive of the authoritative feeding style.

A good friend of mine is a great example of this type of parent. She has mostly healthy food in the house but will offer her child the occasional treat, and when she feeds him at the table, he is not expected to eat what he doesn't want but all the offerings are healthy ones. Her son can choose to eat his chickpeas and broccoli and not touch his whole-grain pasta if he doesn't want to. He is growing up from a very early age with an understanding that healthy food is good for him, and he also knows that he cannot eat treats any time he wants. He sees his mother eating healthy foods all the time, and when dad is around, he tries to be a good role model, too.

Taken to the extreme, these types of parents are the ones who make sandwiches into smiley faces or cut vegetables into cute animal shapes to get their children to eat. But let's be honest, many of us do not have the time to stand on our heads or become artists just to get our children to eat. The good news is that we don't have to go to this extreme.

You do not want to create a situation whereby your children will eat only if there is a fun aspect to their food. By using methods that work—instruction, structure, and encouragement, as well as rules and consequences—you can be running the show without losing your mind. You will learn in chapter 3 exactly what you need to do to remain in control while respecting your children's needs.

The small amount of research that has been done on feeding styles does support that the authoritative feeding style is most effective in bringing up healthy eaters and does make the most sense. How can you go wrong by being firm while taking your children's needs into consideration?

The Spoiler: The Indulgent Parent at the Table

Indulgent parents are warm and nurturing, but they have little oversight or involvement in what their children eat. Indulgent parents put only food they know their children like on their plates to ensure that they finish it. They are not demanding about what food their children eat because their primary focus is on making sure they connect with their children and respond to their needs and desires. An indulgent parent's motivation is one where a positive experience is given priority, and that can mean that children will get what they want and run the show. At the grocery store, indulgent parents buy whatever treats their children want.

The indulgent parent likely believes the current myth that eating and food need to be fun. Indulgent parents are so engaged and focused on an enjoyable experience for their children at the table that it is sometimes (if not usually) to the detriment of their children's diet. If fun is the focus over getting children to eat healthy foods, then what is served looks like this: juice, soda, or chocolate milk to drink, mac 'n' cheese or nuggets dipped in a sweet sauce as a main course, French fries as a side, plus dessert—not vegetables, whole grains, and plain, low-fat milk.

An indulgent feeding style may be the appropriate choice at a birthday party or during vacation, but if it is the daily routine, then children's diets and health will suffer—unless, of course, you have that rare child who loves broccoli and hates sweet foods.

Hands-Off: The Uninvolved Parent at the Table

The truly uninvolved parent has completely backed off at the dinner table. These parents do not monitor their children's food intake, nor do they force or encourage healthy eating. Uninvolved parents allow their children to select their own meals and may not even register whether their children clean their plates. Uninvolved parents have little oversight and are not responsive to their children's needs.

Children of uninvolved parents are most certainly deficient in micronutrients. When it comes to caloric intake, children can just as easily eat too many calories if their diet is based on high-calorie, nutrient-lacking junk or fast food as they can eat too few calories. If their parents have the financial means, the children of uninvolved parents are certainly eating anything they want, which means a diet high in solid fat and added sugar. This type of parenting feeding style is not encouraged.

Which Parenting Style at the Table Is Most Effective?

Over the past twenty years, I have observed that many parents, in an attempt to follow current practices, have let their children's wants supersede their need to make sure their children eat a healthy diet. Many parents I see have an indulgent feeding style because they are fearful that if they push at the table, they will create a child with an eating disorder. Although this fear has a nugget of truth in it, the risks have been widely exaggerated—and at our children's expense.

In conclusion, research suggests that in terms of getting kids to eat a healthy diet, being too overbearing and strict at the table is no better than being too lenient. The authoritative parenting style is the way to go with many other behaviors we teach our children, and even though research is in its infancy, it seems to be the best feeding style as well.

Parent-Centered Quiz: What Is Your Feeding Style?

Did you recognize yourself in any of the feeding styles covered? Did none of them sound like you, or did some behaviors resonate in several of the descriptions? To help you better determine what your feeding style is, complete the quiz below. Answer the questions for each of your children and for how you feed each child in general—not at a party or a restaurant (unless, of course, you eat out more often than you eat in). Circle the number that describes how often these instances occur. If you have a significant other or spouse, have him or her take the quiz, too.

1 Your child must eat his meal at the table. If he does not, you engage in any of the following behaviors (or others not listed) to get him to do so: using physical force, threatening, pleading, begging, or taking away a privilege.

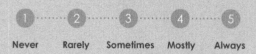

Never   Rarely   Sometimes   Mostly   Always

2 At mealtime or snack time, you usually talk to your child to get her to eat something—saying, for example, "Eat your apple," "Dinner's getting cold," or "Drink your milk because it will make you grow big and strong."

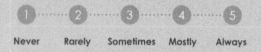

Never   Rarely   Sometimes   Mostly   Always

3 Your child has to stay at the table until he has eaten his food; if he does not, his meal comes back out again or he gets nothing afterward.

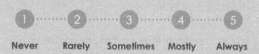

Never   Rarely   Sometimes   Mostly   Always

4 You tell your child to finish the food on her plate or take a certain number of bites before she is allowed to be finished with dinner.

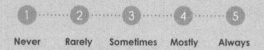

Never   Rarely   Sometimes   Mostly   Always

5 Your child cannot have treats until he has first eaten something healthy.

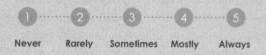

Never   Rarely   Sometimes   Mostly   Always

6 If your child does not eat a certain amount of vegetables or her meal, there is a consequence or reward. For example, you take away a toy or privilege or withhold dessert, or when she does finish, you reward her by allowing her to watch television or get a treat.

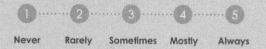

Never   Rarely   Sometimes   Mostly   Always

7 When your child either will not try a bite of a new food or refuses to eat at all, you use any of the following tactics: Tell him to take a bite, reward him for taking a bite, or take away something if he does not take a bite.

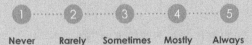

Never   Rarely   Sometimes   Mostly   Always

8 You do not allow certain foods to be served at mealtime or snacks, such as soda, dessert, ketchup, candy, etc.

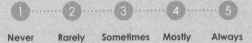

Never   Rarely   Sometimes   Mostly   Always

9 You insist that your child drinks her milk at mealtime or else no dessert, TV, etc., or you reward her with something if she does, such as dessert.

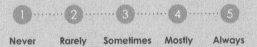

Never   Rarely   Sometimes   Mostly   Always

10 You choose most of the snacks at snack time or the menu at mealtime.

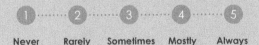

Never   Rarely   Sometimes   Mostly   Always

Add up your total. The scores range from 10 to 50. If your score falls in the 35 to 50 range, then you have an authoritarian or authoritative feeding style. If you scored less than 35, you have either an indulgent or uninvolved feeding style. Take the child-centered quiz next to determine which of the two feeding styles in your range applies to you. Again, answer these questions for each individual child and answer how often these things happen in general.

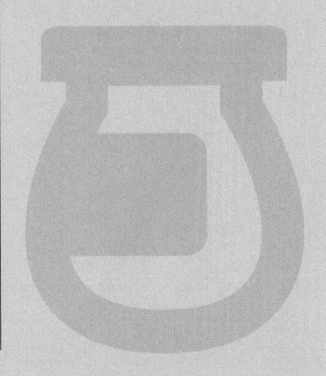

Child-Centered Quiz

1 You give your child choices for snacks or mealtime, such as "Do you want an apple or a banana for snack?" or "Do you want pasta or rice with your chicken?"

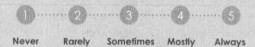

Never   Rarely   Sometimes   Mostly   Always

2 When your child says he is finished eating, you let him leave the table no matter how little he ate. You may ask him "Are you sure?" but that is as far as you will go.

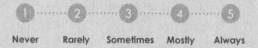

Never   Rarely   Sometimes   Mostly   Always

3 When your child says that she does not like a food, you do not make her try a bite or finish what is on her plate.

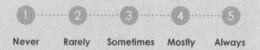

Never   Rarely   Sometimes   Mostly   Always

4 If your child does not want to try a new food, you let it go and do not ask him to take a bite.

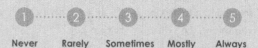

Never   Rarely   Sometimes   Mostly   Always

5 When your child asks for a certain snack at snack time or in the store, you get it for her.

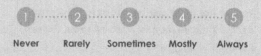

Never   Rarely   Sometimes   Mostly   Always

6 If your child asks for a different meal at mealtime, you cook it for him or let him have a peanut butter and jelly sandwich or other easy-to-fix meal.

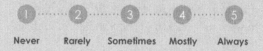

Never   Rarely   Sometimes   Mostly   Always

7 You make smiley face sandwiches or cute shapes out of your child's food to make it fun and engaging for her.

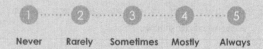

Never   Rarely   Sometimes   Mostly   Always

8 Your child can have as many juice boxes or beverages as he wants.

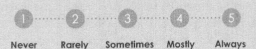

Never   Rarely   Sometimes   Mostly   Always

9 You give your child a snack if she is hungry, even if it is close to mealtime.

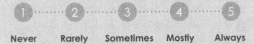

Never   Rarely   Sometimes   Mostly   Always

10 Your child can have as much or as little food as he wants at mealtime or snack time.

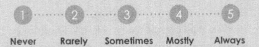

Never   Rarely   Sometimes   Mostly   Always

The scores in the child-centered quiz also range from 10 to 50. Add up your score to see where you fall in this range. If your score falls between 35 and 50, your child has a significant amount of control around food and you have either an authoritative or indulgent feeding style. A score below 35 indicates that your feeding style is either authoritarian or uninvolved. If you take both the scores on the parent and child quizzes and determine where in the table your scores fall, you can determine what feeding style you have.

Score on Parent Control Quiz	Score on Child Control Quiz	Parent Feeding Style
35 to 50	35 to 50	Authoritative
35 to 50	under 35	Authoritarian
under 35	35 to 50	Indulgent
under 35	under 35	Uninvolved

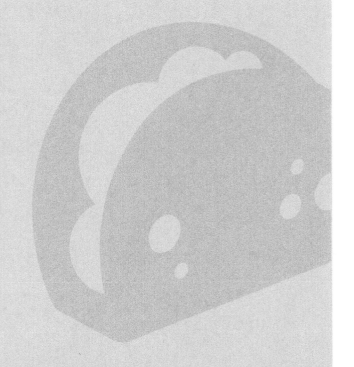

Where Do You Go from Here?

Now that you have determined your and your spouse's feeding style, what's next? To answer this question, it helps to have a better understanding of the inner workings of each feeding style.

Think of these parenting styles as having two dimensions: demandingness and responsiveness. The first dimension, demandingness, is about you, the parent, having control over and supervision of your children (authoritarian, authoritative). This dimension considers your needs. The responsiveness dimension considers the children's needs (indulgent, uninvolved). Responsiveness to your children's needs can include warmth and nurturance toward them if you are an indulgent or authoritative parent. In contrast, the uninvolved and authoritarian feeding style does not take the needs of the child into consideration.

In any relationship, even one between parent and child, when the needs of both parties are considered, it can only be that much better and healthier. Having said that, your goal is to strive for a balance between the two, which is the definition of the authoritative parent. The trick is deciding how much control you, versus your children, need to have. Isn't that the essence of parenting? It is what keeps us up at night; it is what we meet with friends to talk about over coffee; it is what we call our mothers and mothers-in-law about. The amount of control you need versus the amount of control you should give your children will change with their individual personalities and age and the environment. I will go over the balance of control in section 2 with each of the five individual eating personalities; one size does not fit all.

If you and your spouse differ vastly in your parenting styles, you must realize that this is very confusing for children. As a goal, work on getting closer to the authoritative style of parenting, with give-and-take coming from the both of you. No one likes to be told what to do, but if you share this book with your spouse, he or she may well understand why it is so important to create an authoritative parenting style in bringing up healthy eaters and in turning your picky eater around. Who knows, modifying your parenting styles so that they match up closely with the teacher/coach style may change more than food and bring your family closer together as a whole.

Needs Versus Wants

Essential aspects of parenting include love, respect, nurturance, and discipline. The differences between the four feeding styles stem from whose needs are the priority—yours or your children's—and the way you nurture and respect your children.

Because your children do not have the cognitive ability or maturity to understand the complex issues surrounding food, your desires and needs will often be in conflict with theirs. That is obvious, is it not? Although their desires may often run to "I want candy" and "I want soda for dinner," realize that these are wants, not needs. Their need is to eat a healthy diet full of wholesome food and limited in treats, and their desire is the opposite. So while you consider their needs, realize that most often you should not give in to their wants.

Aim for the Authoritative Feeding Style

Now that you have read about the four feeding styles, you may have found that you are definitely one type, or you may have discovered that you practice one or two styles depending on the situation. The parent with an indulgent feeding style may feel good giving his or her child what the child wants, but it is often not what the child needs to grow up strong and healthy. The uninvolved style—well, that never leads to anything good. Kids are not supposed to parent themselves—that is what we are here for. The take-home message is that most of the time being a teacher or coach is the way to go.

In addition, as mentioned previously, what works for one child may not work for another. On the parent-involvement scale, you may need to be closer to one end than the other depending on what works best for your specific child. You may, and most likely do, have different eaters who show up to your table. I do: With one child, I have needed to monitor and intervene in his diet very little. He always ate what was given to him without much fuss. My little one, however, needs constant monitoring or he would be off and running down junk-food alley in a heartbeat.

The way you interact with each of your eaters will consist of a number of behaviors that you display around food. In the next chapter, you will learn which of these feeding practices are essential for making you an effective teacher and coach and which ones do not. You will discover which feeding practices have a positive outcome, which ones depend on the specific situation, and which ones to avoid.

CHAPTER 2

Discover Feeding Practices that Work for Your Child

In this chapter, you will learn about feeding practices that are essential for turning around a picky eater and how to establish and reinforce healthy eating behaviors. The practices and behaviors listed pertain not just to the picky eater, but to all children who have a difficult time eating enough of the recommended foods they need each day: fruits, vegetables, whole grains, and healthy sources of protein and fat.

You will be asked to take a quiz in each of the three parts of this chapter to determine how often you engage in these practices and behaviors. Once you know which feeding practices you excel at, which ones need improvement, and which ones you need to learn, you will be well on your way to not only creating healthy eaters but keeping them that way. You may need to complete a quiz for each of your children if you or they interact differently around food or if they vary in age.

Some of the following feeding behaviors, such as mirroring healthy eating, are great for everyone to practice, whether or not you're dealing with a picky eater. Other practices, such as monitoring eating habits, will depend on your child's eating personality, age, and other factors. Finally, others, such as using force to get a child to eat, should be avoided. Find out which feeding practices you currently engage in and to what degree.

1. Rate Yourself: Feeding Practices that Work

This information will determine which beneficial feeding practices you currently engage in and to what degree. The five practices listed here will form your toolbox for creating a healthy eater: mirror healthy eating, make sure you have healthy food at home, teach your children why they need to eat a healthy diet, encourage them to do so, and involve them in the selection and cooking of healthy food.

Mirroring Healthy Eating

When a son sees his dad shave and imitates the shaving motion with his finger, that is mirroring. When a little girl carries a pocketbook and wants to try on high heels after watching her mom head off to work dressed to the nines, that is mirroring. When your son wants soda or gobbles down ice cream when he is feeling angry, that may be mirroring if you do the same. If your daughter never sees you eating fresh vegetables, chances are she won't eat them either. Learn how your dietary practices affect your children's eating habits by taking the first quiz.

The following questions ask about *your* diet and eating practices.

1. **How much of your daily diet is made up of healthy food (at least three vegetables, two fruits, whole grains, and healthy protein and fats)?**

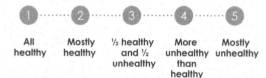

| All healthy | Mostly healthy | ½ healthy and ½ unhealthy | More unhealthy than healthy | Mostly unhealthy |

2. **How often do you eat or drink treats and junk foods (cakes, cookies, soda, candy, chips, etc.)?**

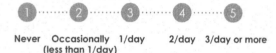

| Never | Occasionally (less than 1/day) | 1/day | 2/day | 3/day or more |

3. **Do you tend to use food to help you deal with stress or your emotions?**

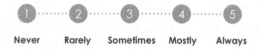

| Never | Rarely | Sometimes | Mostly | Always |

4. **Do you tend to eat past being full?**

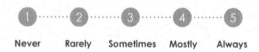

| Never | Rarely | Sometimes | Mostly | Always |

Your actions at the table are more important than what you say when it comes to being a food role model. Research is clear that modeling of eating habits has a very strong influence on children's eating behaviors. Your children are learning more than just *what* they should eat, they are learning *how* to eat. For example, do they eat when they are upset? Do they eat quickly and absent-mindedly while watching television? Will they go for dessert even though they didn't eat much at dinner?

Let's check how well you do with modeling your eating behaviors for your children. Add up your score and find the range where it lands below.

4 to 8: GREAT JOB!

You are doing a wonderful job modeling healthy eating for your children. It is the single most effective tool you have as a parent to teach your children how to eat healthy. Note: If you scored a 4 or higher on any of the questions above, try working on that behavior until you can get it down to a 1 or 2.

9 to 15: YOU ARE ON YOUR WAY.

However, you need to focus on some of your eating habits. Make healthy eating a family affair and work on it together, especially in the areas where you scored a 4 or more on.

16 to 20: YOU NEED HELP!

You will need to work on your eating habits while you work on your children's. Younger children especially watch everything you do and tend to copy it. As your children get older, their peers will have more of an influence, but you will always have an effect on them. You also deserve to live a healthy life no matter how stressed you are, and a healthy diet is part of that.

I know that it can be overwhelming to have to focus on *your* diet right now while you are struggling to get your child to eat a healthy diet. The thought of eating healthier may be too much for you. I understand, which is why I developed an eating plan that focuses on the busy family. At my site, www.buildhealthykids.com, you will focus on making one change at a time—that way, your family can make one step toward health each month together. You can also use all the tools and information you will learn in this book to help you make that change.

Access to Healthy Foods

1 Do you usually have healthy food in the house (e.g., fresh fruit and vegetables, whole grains, low-fat dairy products, and healthy sources of protein)?

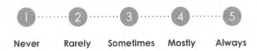

Never   Rarely   Sometimes   Mostly   Always

2 Are fresh fruit and vegetables in reach and easy for your child to access?

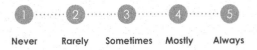

Never   Rarely   Sometimes   Mostly   Always

3 Circle the amount of sweet or salty treats (e.g., chips, candy, soda, cookies, or cake) you normally keep in the house at any given time.

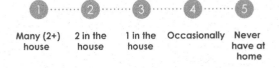

Many (2+) house   2 in the house   1 in the house   Occasionally   Never have at home

4 Do you keep soda, sports drinks, flavored water, flavored milk, or energy drinks in the house?

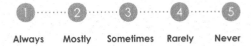

Always   Mostly   Sometimes   Rarely   Never

Having healthy food and beverages in your house makes healthy eating a whole lot easier, especially when things get crazy and rushed at home. Keeping a well-stocked pantry and shopping on the weekend for the week ahead to make sure you have fresh and healthy foods on hand will set you up to serve some great-tasting, good-for-you meals and snacks throughout the week.

However, having too much unhealthy food and beverages in the house will promote unhealthy eating habits. As a nutritionist and a mom whose kids love treats as much as the next, I usually have only one treat option in the house at a time. Some parents go so far as to forbid any type of junk food in the house, but I know that doing this will cause my boys to crave more of it. Research shows that forbidding food may cause your children to desire more of the food you restrict. It is better to have a little bit on hand that is offered infrequently than to forbid a certain food or drink.

See how well you scored on access to healthy food. Add up your scores on questions 1 through 4 above and read the information below that corresponds to your score.

16 to 20: GREAT JOB!

You are doing a wonderful job making sure that your child has access to healthy food and that unhealthy food is limited. Note: If you scored a 2 or lower on any of the questions above, work on that behavior until you can get it up to a 4 or 5.

9 to 15: YOU ARE ON YOUR WAY.

However, try to get more healthy food into and more unhealthy food out of the house. Work on replacing an unhealthy food with a healthy alternative, one food at a time. For example, replace gummy fruit snacks with whole fruit or soda with flavored unsweetened seltzer water. Too much change at once is likely to backfire.

4 to 8: YOU NEED HELP.

Here are ways to make healthy foods more accessible in your household:

- Start by purchasing fresh fruits and vegetables. This is the single most important change you can do. These items are essential to have on hand for your child to snack on and for you to add to a meal.

- Grab some healthy protein options (e.g., nuts, low-fat yogurt, or cheese) and whole grains (e.g., whole grain bread, crackers, and breakfast items).

- Replace each unhealthy food with a healthy one until you have made the switch to mostly healthy food and limited junk food. For example, substitute low-fat cheese sticks for cheese out of a can, then replace chocolate milk with plain low-fat milk.

Be ready: Your children will throw a fit the first time they look for a juice box or candy in the cabinet and it isn't there. But once they get used to it, they will look for other options. The trick is being consistent. If you give in now and again, it will take much, much longer to establish a new habit—in fact, if you're not consistent, it may never happen. The key is keeping handy, healthy, easy-to-grab foods and snack options in the house, such as nuts, dried fruit, fresh fruit and vegetables, yogurt cups, whole-grain crackers or pretzels, and cheese sticks.

Teaching Nutrition to Kids

1 **Do you teach your children why they need to eat healthy food?**

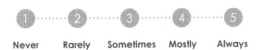

Never   Rarely   Sometimes   Mostly   Always

2 **Do you teach your children about the health benefits of healthy food and the ill effects of unhealthy food?**

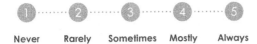

Never   Rarely   Sometimes   Mostly   Always

3 **When you go shopping with your child or order out, do you explain which foods are healthy and which ones are not?**

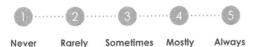

Never   Rarely   Sometimes   Mostly   Always

4 **If you cook with your children, do you explain which ingredients are healthy and which ones are not?**

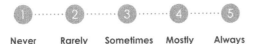

Never   Rarely   Sometimes   Mostly   Always

Today's feeding recommendations need to catch up to the current food environment, which is what *The Picky Eating Solution* is all about. Long gone are the days where we worked from sun up to sun down and our only food choices were right outside our front door or within our neighborhood. Because our neighborhoods are now made up of tasty, cheap, and easy-to-find unhealthy items, we need to teach children how and why they need to eat a diet rich in healthy choices.

The basic foundation of this teaching is *almost everything straight from nature is good for us while processed items need to be limited or avoided.* Our children need to learn that:

- The majority of their diet needs to consist of healthy food.

- Unhealthy foods need to be an occasional treat.

- Liquids should be almost exclusively water or milk.

- They also need to know why this way of eating is necessary: "Because you'll grow up big and strong if you eat this" is most often enough of an explanation for younger children, and "Because this food is needed for you to reach your potential and stay healthy" is a start for the older child.

Determine how well you did on instructing your children on why they need to eat a healthy diet and limit junk. Add up items 1 through 4 above and see where your score falls below.

16 to 20: GREAT JOB!

You are doing a fantastic job using daily opportunities to teach children how to select healthy foods and why doing so is important. Note: If you scored a 2 or lower on any of these 4 questions, work on that behavior until you can get it up to a 4 or 5.

9 to 15: YOU ARE ON YOUR WAY.

However, use more opportunities to teach your children how to eat healthfully. Eating a healthy diet now takes knowledge because the majority of our food options are processed. You need to tell children why you are selecting certain foods and not others at the store or for a recipe. Work on those areas that you scored a 2 or lower on.

4 to 8: YOU NEED HELP.

Just like children need to know why they have to look both ways before crossing the street, they need to know why they need to eat their vegetables and why they can't survive on candy and soda. If you need help with what to teach your child, my website, www.buildhealthykids.com, will provide that information for you. You can also check out other nutrition programs and websites in the Resources section of the book to help you teach your child nutrition essentials.

Encouraging Healthy Eating Habits

1 Do you encourage your children to eat healthy food or praise them when they do?

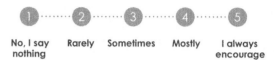

No, I say nothing   Rarely   Sometimes   Mostly   I always encourage

2 Do you encourage your children to eat healthy food first before they eat their treat (e.g., apple before cookie, cheese before chips)?

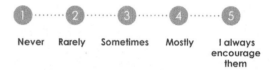

Never   Rarely   Sometimes   Mostly   I always encourage them

3 Do you praise your children when they do a good job eating an appropriate portion of healthy food?

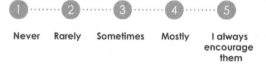

Never   Rarely   Sometimes   Mostly   I always encourage them

If your children do not eat a healthy diet or eat too much junk food, then your goal is to score a 4 or more on each of these questions. Once your child starts to master eating healthy and limiting snacks, you can drop your encouragement a little bit at a time. It doesn't hurt to praise anyone now and again though, even an older child or spouse: "Great job stopping at one bowl of ice cream, your stomach will thank you for that later."

Where praise and encouragement is usually needed is at the table when your children take one bite of food, say they are done, and then ask for dessert. You need to know what appropriate serving sizes are for your child so you have reasonable expectations at mealtime. For example, you'd expect a three-year-old to eat three spears of broccoli versus a ½ cup (36 g) for an eight-year old. Chapter 4 has lists of typical serving sizes for children of all ages and techniques to help you determine whether your children are really full when they say they are.

Once your children have mastered a task, there is no reason to continue to praise them about it all the time. I no longer have to say "Great job brushing your teeth" to my ten-year-old, for example. You can tone down the "Wow, you ate all of your broccoli. That is fantastic!" when your children have mastered doing the task independently of your praise.

By praising good behavior, you encourage that behavior, plain and simple. When you praise your children for eating healthy food and limiting unhealthy food, you are encouraging both of these behaviors to happen again and again. For some children, you can be subtle about it, but for others—well, get out the pom-poms. Certain eating personalities need more encouragement than others, and you will be guided as to who needs more and who needs less in section 2.

Involving Your Child in All Things Food Related

1 **How often do you bring your child into the kitchen to help you cook or prepare meals (includes interacting and observing for the very young)?**

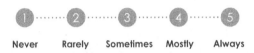

Never   Rarely   Sometimes   Mostly   Always

2 **How often do you bring your child grocery shopping with you?**

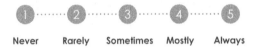

Never   Rarely   Sometimes   Mostly   Always

3 **How often do you sit down as a family and eat a meal together?**

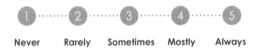

Never   Rarely   Sometimes   Mostly   Always

4 **How often do you bring your children to a farm, farmers market, or vegetable garden to show them how food is grown (includes growing plants in your window box, terrace, community garden, or home garden)?**

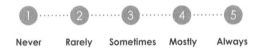

Never   Rarely   Sometimes   Mostly   Always

To find out how well you involve your children in all things food related, add up your scores. Find the range that your score falls within below.

16 to 20: GREAT JOB!

You are exposing your children to critical information and developing their skills when it comes to choosing and preparing food. Keep up the good work and grow with your children: Allow them to prepare more of the meal as they get older and give them more responsibility in the grocery store. Note: If you scored a 2 or lower on any of the 4 questions above, work on that behavior until you can get it up to a 4 or 5.

9 to 15: YOU ARE ON YOUR WAY.

As much as you may not like to bring your children shopping or involve them in cooking because they will be in your way in the kitchen, it is important to do these activities. Set ground rules first: They must behave or they leave the kitchen, or you both leave the store. In the grocery store, have them select fresh produce, look for the expiration date on the milk, and hunt for whole grains. In the kitchen, give them busy work to do while you prepare dinner. The sink can provide endless fascination for young children, for example. Specifically work on those areas on which you scored a 2 or lower.

4 to 8: WARNING.

You need to start getting your children more involved in food-related activities. You do not want them growing up with no knowledge of how to identify food, where it comes from, or the impact their selections have on their body. Try these suggestions:

- Start slowly. Consider bringing them shopping with you once a week. Start at the produce aisle and have them select some oranges, for example.

- If your children tend to whine and plead in the store, give them the privilege of selecting their one treat for the week. If they whine, that treat goes back on the shelf, and they lose that privilege for the week. You will be surprised how fast they will behave after that.

- Get them involved. Treat grocery shopping as if it were a scavenger hunt. For older children, make them responsible for a part of your grocery list. For younger children, stay with them and have them find the cereal among the dozens of options before you.

- In the kitchen, start off slowly as well. Have them wash fruits and vegetables or find ingredients in the cupboard or pantry for you.

- Remember to praise them for the little steps that they take and give yourself a pat on the back, too. I know how busy your life can be, and taking the time to teach your children how to eat healthfully gives them an essential skill, but it is also a sacrifice on your time. It's worth it, though!

Children who have exposure to farms or local farmers markets or who grow things in their home or neighborhood are learning more than how to garden. They are learning where food comes from, plus what it looks like in its whole form. These kids wouldn't call a piece of pizza a vegetable or believe that a glow-in-the-dark candy came from the earth. Many children have limited knowledge on how to identify fresh fruits and vegetables and are grossed out when they find that they grow out of the dirt. Getting children back into nature will help them to discover that chicken does not come in convenient nugget shapes, milk does not come out of the cow chocolate flavored and in boxes, and potatoes do not grow in small strips that just need to be heated up.

As inconvenient as it may seem, having your children assist you in the kitchen is critical for them. They are learning, like every other mammal on this planet does in the wild, what to do with the food they need to survive. Preparing food starts with asking their input on menu selections: "What vegetable do you want to eat with the chicken tonight?" for example. Younger children will naturally sniff, touch, and maybe even taste food that they are measuring or washing. My son started eating raw broccoli like it was a lollipop when he washed it in the sink, around the fourth time he interacted with it. Children need to know their food before trusting it and sometimes even before they will taste it. This takes repeated exposure.

We have all heard the saying "Bring a man a fish and you have fed him for one day; teach a man to fish and you have taught him how to feed himself for life." The same holds true for our children: Swinging by fast-food restaurants and pulling up to the window does not show them how to sort through the unhealthy options to find the healthy ones, nor does just putting dinner down in front of them with no knowledge of where it came from.

2. Rate Yourself: Feeding Practices that Vary

A one-size-fits-all approach does not work when it comes to monitoring and controlling what your children eat. The amount of monitoring and control can change according to the following:

- **Different situations.** You may not need to supervise your children's food intake at home, but at a restaurant they need to be monitored because they are so distracted with the frenzy of the setting and all those choices. An example of a time when you let things slide might be when a friend is over and children are off the walls with excitement.

- **Current diet quality.** The degree of monitoring and control you exert will depend on your children's diet—specifically the amount of healthy food they consume each day. At the beginning of the process of turning around picky eaters, for example, you will need to oversee and control much more than you will once they master eating their vegetables.

- **Age.** All children—no matter their age—need some degree of monitoring. The trick is to be subtler about it with your older children. Younger children will need more supervision in general than older children, but some older children have diets that are so unhealthy that you will need to monitor them more closely and exert greater control more than you would for another child their age. In addition to making sure that your very young children get all the nutritional requirements they need, you also need to monitor them to make sure they are eating correctly to prevent choking.

After the age of six, picky eating decreases as the child gets older and remains stable in adulthood until old age, when it appears to rise again.

People go through periods of highs and lows of biologically driven states of picky eating. In one review of picky eating and neophobia (the fear of eating new foods), researchers determined the general consensus is that children go through a period of increased picky eating and fear of unknown foods that peaks between the ages two and six. After the age of six, picky eating decreases as the child gets older and remains stable in adulthood until old age, when it appears to rise again ("Food Neophobia and 'Picky/Fussy' Eating in Children: A Review," Terence M. Dovey et al. *Appetite* 50 [2008] 181–193). The degrees of control and monitoring during these phases should follow the pattern outlined earlier, and in times of heightened pickiness, control and monitoring need to be increased. The following factors also influence the level of monitoring and contact:

- **Physical or emotional limitations.** If your children have a physical or emotional disability, such as ADHD, autism, or cystic fibrosis, they will need much more monitoring and control than children without these conditions. Children with these types of conditions will need personal guidance from a professional close to home, such as an occupational therapist or nutritionist, for example. Whereas most children will give in and finally eat a meal even if it is not what they want, children with physical or emotional limitations may not.

- **The physical and emotional environment.** Eating at a restaurant versus eating at home will require more monitoring and control, especially for younger children. They will be tempted with all the unhealthy options on the menu, and they know that they can get away with things in public that they may not be able to at home. If there are guests at the table or a sibling is having a bad day, the degree of encouragement and monitoring will also vary.

Monitoring Your Children's Diet

1   **In general, how much do you pay attention to your child's intake of food and drink?**

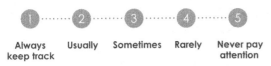

| Always keep track | Usually | Sometimes | Rarely | Never pay attention |

2   **Do you keep track of the amount of unhealthy junk food (e.g., soda, desserts, sweets, and chips) that your child eats?**

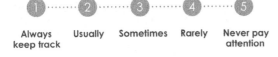

| Always keep track | Usually | Sometimes | Rarely | Never pay attention |

3   **Do you monitor the amount of healthy food that your child eats?**

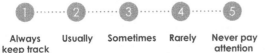

| Always keep track | Usually | Sometimes | Rarely | Never pay attention |

4   **Do you monitor your child's intake of food and beverages eaten away from home (e.g., at school, at parties, or on playdates)?**

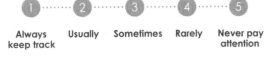

| Always keep track | Usually | Sometimes | Rarely | Never pay attention |

Add up your scores for questions 1 through 4 and find your range below:

16 to 20: LIGHT MONITORING.

This degree of monitoring is appropriate for children who eat their daily requirements independently and without much fuss. If you are in this category, you are occasionally monitoring your children's eating, checking in to make sure everything is still as it should be.

However, because you are dealing with a picky eater, chances are good that your child is not independently eating what he needs to each day, so you need to increase the amount of monitoring that you currently do. Once your child eats more healthy foods, you can slowly begin to decrease the amount of monitoring. For now, though, shoot for "usually" or "always" keeping track of their intake.

9 to 15: MEDIUM MONITORING.

If your children's diet is made up of mostly healthy food and the occasional treat, then you are doing a great job with monitoring. Chances are, however, that this is not the case because you're dealing with a picky eater. Increase your level of monitoring to one where you are usually checking on their intake. For most picky eaters, a medium degree of monitoring is usually needed throughout their childhood because these types of eaters tend to slip back into old ways of eating as soon as they have an opportunity.

Monitoring does not need to be a full-time job. Consider the following a typical day of monitoring, which is sufficient in bringing up healthy eaters:

A change in eating habits is a sign that you need to pay more attention to your child.

- **Breakfast:** Look to see what your picky eater ate and didn't eat. Encourage her to eat more if she just ate a couple of bites or pack the rest of her meal to eat on the way to school or sports. Because breakfast is essential for fueling her mind and body for school, encourage her to eat even if she is not hungry at 6 or 7 a.m. Make a smoothie with yogurt, fruit, and a dash of milk or juice to get your child going.

- **Lunch:** Pack a lunch for your child or check what he packed. When he gets home from school, casually ask whether he ate his meal: "Did you like lunch today? Were you able to eat it all?" or if your child buys lunch, "What did you buy for lunch today? Was it good? Did you finish it? Would you order it again?"

- **Snack:** If you are home, observe what your child eats for a snack. If you do not like what you see, say, "Those cookies are a yummy option for snack. Why don't you get a fruit to go with them?" For the older child, ask "Were you able to get something to eat after school? What was it?" Armed with this information, you are able to design dinner to fill in the gaps. If your child didn't consume enough vegetables or milk, serve two veggies for dinner and make sure she drinks a glass of milk with them. If your child's fruit requirement for the day was not met, serve fruit— or if she's had too many treats, serve fruit as the only dessert.

4 to 8: HEAVY MONITORING.

You currently monitor your child's intake most of the time. For very picky eaters, this is necessary until their diet improves. Depending on your child's eating personality, you may or may not need to adjust your level of monitoring (you will learn more about that in section 2). The degree of monitoring you do also depends on what you do with what you observe. Just because you are watching what your children eat does not mean that you are doing something about it. If you take the information that you learned from your observations and become militant about your child's diet, then that is not in anyone's best interest. In the next part of this chapter on control, you will learn what to do with your observations.

No matter what kind of diet your child follows, some observation is needed to assess whether your child's appetite is changing. Children go through so many physical and emotional stages as they age that one of the best tools you have to gauge their health by is observing their eating habits. An increased appetite may mean that they are going through a growth spurt or that they are stressed and using food to soothe themselves. Not eating enough food may be a sign that things are off or it could be due to a natural decrease during their childhood. Either way, a change in eating habits is a sign that you need to pay more attention to your child. Ask her how she is feeling or whether something happened recently that upset her. If things do not improve or you are still concerned, seek the advice of their pediatrician.

Control Over Your Child's Diet

I believe that control is the most hotly debated and misunderstood feeding practice. *Control* can be a heated word in the nutrition community, but when you look into it, it is a practice that can take on characteristics ranging from encouragement to force. Like any other behavior, *how* you practice is as important as *what* you practice. Control can be done adversely with a Mr./Mrs. Strict approach or in a way that is pleasing to children through a Teacher/Coach approach. The next twenty questions will determine where you land on the control scale.

1 **My child chooses his own snack.**

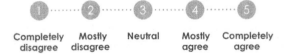

2 **I decide which foods my child should have at snack time.**

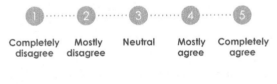

3 **I decide when my child can have a snack.**

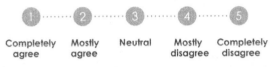

4 **My child can get a snack anytime she wants to.**

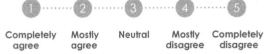

5 **I pack my child's lunch or select the lunch he can buy at school.**

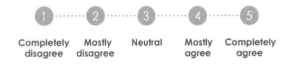

6 **My child has to taste at least one bite of a new food.**

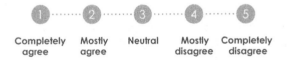

7 **If my child does not want to try a new food, I do not encourage or force her to.**

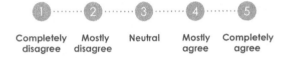

8   I let my children choose which foods to have
     at mealtime. They can choose as much of one
     food as they want and leave off the vegetables,
     for example.

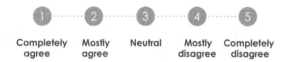

| Completely agree | Mostly agree | Neutral | Mostly disagree | Completely disagree |

9   I serve my child at mealtime: I choose what
     and how much food he will eat and place it on
     his plate.

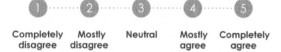

| Completely disagree | Mostly disagree | Neutral | Mostly agree | Completely agree |

10   My child gets to select the beverage she wants
     at mealtime.

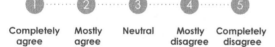

| Completely agree | Mostly agree | Neutral | Mostly disagree | Completely disagree |

11   I choose the beverages at mealtime.

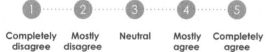

| Completely disagree | Mostly disagree | Neutral | Mostly agree | Completely agree |

12   My child can drink as much as he wants
     at mealtime.

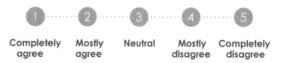

| Completely agree | Mostly agree | Neutral | Mostly disagree | Completely disagree |

13   I make sure that my child is eating enough at
     mealtime before I let her have a refill on her
     beverage.

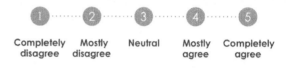

| Completely disagree | Mostly disagree | Neutral | Mostly agree | Completely agree |

14   I let my child decide how much of his meal he
     wants to eat.

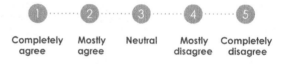

| Completely agree | Mostly agree | Neutral | Mostly disagree | Completely disagree |

15   I make sure that my child has eaten an
     appropriate portion of her meal; if not, I either
     serve it later or I won't let her be excused until
     she finishes.

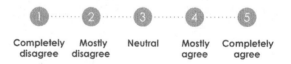

| Completely disagree | Mostly disagree | Neutral | Mostly agree | Completely agree |

16 My child cannot have dessert if he hasn't eaten enough dinner.

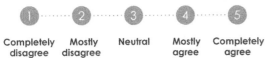

| Completely disagree | Mostly disagree | Neutral | Mostly agree | Completely agree |

17 My children can have dessert no matter what they ate for dinner.

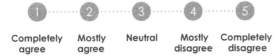

| Completely agree | Mostly agree | Neutral | Mostly disagree | Completely disagree |

18 When grocery shopping, my child can select any type of food or beverage that she wants.

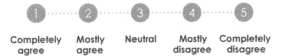

| Completely agree | Mostly agree | Neutral | Mostly disagree | Completely disagree |

19 My child can eat whatever he wants after dinner even though he may have eaten little for dinner.

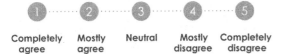

| Completely agree | Mostly agree | Neutral | Mostly disagree | Completely disagree |

20 I make most, if not all, the selections at the grocery store.

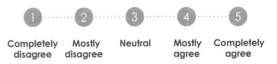

| Completely disagree | Mostly disagree | Neutral | Mostly agree | Completely agree |

Add up your score from questions 1 through 20 above. Your score will range from 20 to 100. The closer you score to 100, the more control you have over your child's eating behaviors; the closer you score to 20, the more your child has control over his or her food and beverage choices. A score of 60 reflects a situation where both of you have equal control.

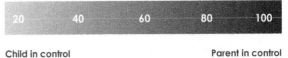

Child in control   Parent in control

Where should you land on this scale? There is no one correct answer except to not fall on either extreme— giving your child total control (indulgent) or forcing him to eat (authoritarian). Unlike the other feeding practices listed previously, there are no score ranges that are specific goals for you to reach. The amount of control you have over your child differs depending on many factors—some are listed in this chapter and others are summarized in section 2, where you will learn how much control your child needs based on his or her temperament and eating personality.

When force enters into the equation and fear is the result, leave the table.

- **Your child's *ability* to select healthy food.** Young children or children with certain mental or physical disorders will not have the cognitive ability to make healthy choices, so we as parents need to step in and make these decisions for them. In these situations, it is still important to give children choices, but make both options healthy ones. There are also many older children who have not been taught the difference between healthy food and treats. With this age group, start by educating them on the differences between the two and serve mostly healthy choices until they understand which are healthy. For children who have emotional issues or lie anywhere on the autism spectrum, control can be a tricky thing. Whereas I would advise the parents of picky eaters to excuse their children from dinner if they did not finish and offer the food to them again later, children with autism or taste aversion may not come back later or ever to finish their food.

- **Your child's *willingness* to select healthy food.** Just because your child is capable of making healthy choices does not mean that he will. This is where your child needs to earn your trust, just like in many other areas of his life. You wouldn't let your child walk to the end of the block until you saw that she knew how to cross the street and wouldn't walk into traffic. The same holds true for eating: Don't let your child have too much control until you have observed that he not only *can* but *will* make healthy choices the majority of time.

- **Your child's personality.** All children need you to be in charge to some degree, even though they may not like it. The way you exert control, however, will be vastly different when you are dealing with strong-willed children versus easygoing ones. You do not need to hide your control as much with easygoing children as you would with strong-willed children.

- **Your child's health.** If your child is ill or suffers from a chronic disease such as diabetes, you need to have more control over her eating behaviors than you would for a child who is healthy. The same holds true for children who are at risk of developing diseases, including those who are overweight or obese.

  NOTE: It is *never* okay to put your child on a diet without strict medical supervision. Children need to get enough nutrients to grow and reach their potential, and by restricting food, you could and most likely would prevent this from happening. The focus should also *never* be on weight, but always on health.

- **Your child's age.** The degree of control you have in any situation will diminish as your child gets older and demonstrates mastery of a certain task. Your ultimate goal as a parent is to send your child out of the house with the ability to do the following:

- Know the difference between healthy and unhealthy food

- Understand why it is essential to eat a diet full of healthy food choices and why treats need to be limited

- Identify at the grocery store which foods are healthy and which are not

- Know where real food comes from

- Know how to cook at least five meals on his or her own

- Know where to find information, recipes, and advice about food when necessary

This discussion would not be complete unless I spoke about force. Forcing children to eat is never okay in any situation. This is control taken to the extreme, and it is abusive, plain and simple. When force enters into the equation and fear is the result, leave the table. In these situations, it is best to give yourself a time out and show yourself some compassion because you most likely learned this behavior by being forced to eat at some point in your life. It is time to learn another way, and that is what I am here to teach you.

Creating consequences is as far as you should take your attempts to get children to eat, and the next chapter will describe setting rules and consequences in detail.

NOTE: Parents of children with autism and other disabilities sometimes use force as the last resort before tube feedings are necessary, but even in these situations force is never a good thing. Instead, seek professional help from someone who works with children on the spectrum.

Restricting Certain Foods

Left to their own devices, children would eat mostly junk food. Our job as parents is to know when and by how much to restrict these unhealthy options in their diet. Find out where you are on the restriction scale.

1 **How often do you allow your child to eat cookies, cake, candy, and other treats?**

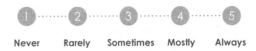

Never   Rarely   Sometimes   Mostly   Always

2 **Do you keep treats in the house?**

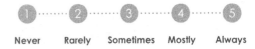

Never   Rarely   Sometimes   Mostly   Always

3 **Do you restrict the amount of sweets, desserts, and other junk food that your child can have in a day?**

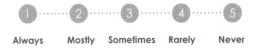

Always   Mostly   Sometimes   Rarely   Never

4 **Do you restrict the amount of soda or juice that your child can have in a day?**

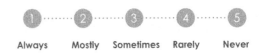

Always   Mostly   Sometimes   Rarely   Never

Add up your score from questions 1 through 4 to see your results.

4 to 6: TOO RESTRICTIVE.

If you completely restrict treats in and out of your house, you may be creating a situation in which your children will crave them and eat more of them when they do get their hands on them—at least that is what some research suggests, although the findings are not consistent.

7 to 12: A HAPPY MEDIUM.

As long as you did not score a 4 or 5 on questions 1, 3, or 4, you have reached a great balance. It is all right to have some treats in the house as long as you manage how much is consumed on a daily basis; one a day is a good limit.

13 to 20: NOT RESTRICTIVE ENOUGH.

If you scored a 13 or above, it means that you allow your child to eat too many treats. Try to limit treats to one per day on most days. You may need to remove some from the house if they are too tempting. Keep one type on hand until you have things under control.

The majority (85 to 90 percent) of children's food needs to be healthy; a once-a-day treat is fine for healthy children.

Too much sugar, however, in children's diets can lead to the following:

- ADHD and other learning and behavioral disorders
- Anxiety and depression
- Bone fractures
- Cavities
- Candidiasis (yeast infection)
- Chronic fatigue syndrome and fibromyalgia
- Chronic sinusitis and ear infections
- Decreased immune function and increased susceptibility to infections and serious diseases such as cancer
- Diabetes
- Heart disease
- Irritable bowel syndrome and spastic colon
- Metabolic syndrome

Using Food as a Reward

Using food as a reward has received the most media attention when compared to other eating practices. Find out whether and how you use food as a reward by taking the following quiz.

1 **Do you reward your child with food or beverages when he has a non-food-related achievement (e.g., if he gets an A on a test, he gets a candy bar; if she learns to ride her bike, she gets an ice cream cone; or a soccer win scores him a piece of cake)?**

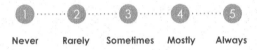

Never　Rarely　Sometimes　Mostly　Always

2 **Do you withhold treats from your child if she behaves badly?**

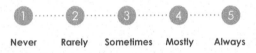

Never　Rarely　Sometimes　Mostly　Always

3 **Do you give your child a specific food or beverage if he completes a food-related activity that he doesn't want to do (e.g., finishing dinner gets him dessert, eating her fruit gets her a cookie, eating his vegetables gets him ice cream, or finishing her milk gets her another helping of French fries)?**

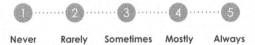

Never　Rarely　Sometimes　Mostly　Always

4 **Do your children have to eat something healthy before they can have a treat?**

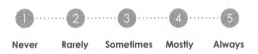

Never　Rarely　Sometimes　Mostly　Always

Questions 1 and 2 above are very similar, as are questions 3 and 4. This is intentional because I like to separate out the true essence of *reward* from that of *consequence*. Giving a food treat when your child wins a game, aces a test, or performs well on stage is using food to reward a desirable behavior. Not allowing dessert until enough dinner is eaten, especially vegetables, is a consequence, *not* a reward. So is having your child eat the healthy stuff before he can have the unhealthy part of his snack. This is really just a "this then that" technique you probably use every day, whereby you teach your child that he must first do one thing before he can get what he wants: exercise before playing video games, finish homework before playing outside, or clean up your room before going to a friend's house. If you take away the consequence, how in the world are you ever going to motivate your child to eat the healthy stuff?

If your score from questions 1 and 2 adds up to between 8 and 10, you are using food as a reward for non-food-related activities too often in your child's diet. If, however, the added score of questions 3 and 4 are within the 8 and 10 range, then you are using food appropriately to promote healthy eating.

The following are examples of when using food as a reward or rewarding healthful eating is fine:

- It is used occasionally in a family where healthy food is the norm and unhealthy food is allowed occasionally. In this type of feeding environment, children learn that they have to focus on the healthy stuff and limit the unhealthy stuff.

- It is used to get a very stubborn picky eater to eat a food he otherwise would not: if your picky eater tries the broccoli, he can have an extra 15 minutes for electronics, for example. Use this approach with caution and for only the beginning two or three exposures to a certain food because you do not want to teach your child that he always gets more electronic time when he eats what he is supposed to in the first place.

- It is not used with children who are junk-food junkies. The sweet treat reward will just aggravate their cravings for more sweets.

- It is not used with children who have weight issues, diabetes, or other physical or mental conditions that are negatively affected by sweets.

- It is reserved for rewarding major accomplishments and not for the day-to-day advances our children make. Kids love praise and attention, so shower them with that instead of with sugar.

3. Rate Yourself: Feeding Practices to Avoid

Because food has a pleasurable aspect to it, many of us eat not because we have to but because we want to. This hedonistic quality of food can be used to soothe our emotions or help us just feel better when we are stressed. On one extreme, food can be used as a drug like any other to manage our crazy lives, and for many people, sugar is addictive. (My previous book, *Beat Sugar Addiction Now! for Kids*, discusses that topic in depth.) For others, food can be pleasurable but it doesn't rule their life; it is an afterthought. Determine where you are in feeding your child's emotions with food by taking the next quiz.

Emotional Feeding

1 **My child loves food, especially treats and junk food.**

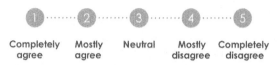

Completely agree · Mostly agree · Neutral · Mostly disagree · Completely disagree

2 **I use food to help my child feel better when he is stressed, upset, or just had a bad day.**

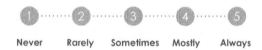

Never · Rarely · Sometimes · Mostly · Always

3 **When my child is sick, I give her treats or her favorite food to make her feel better.**

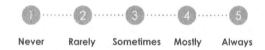

Never · Rarely · Sometimes · Mostly · Always

4 **I use food to connect with my child (e.g., we go out for ice cream or I sit and have cookies and milk with him) or to show love.**

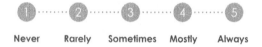

Never · Rarely · Sometimes · Mostly · Always

Add up your scores from questions 2, 3, and 4 (we'll get to question 1 in a minute) to determine where you are on the emotional feeding scale. If you scored 12 to 15 points (or if you scored a 4 or 5 on any one of the questions), you typically use food to make your children feel better. A score between 7 and 11 means you sometimes use food to soothe emotions, and a score of 6 or below means you do not usually use food to manage your child's emotions.

What this means for your individual child really depends on how rewarding food is for him or her. If your child scored a 4 or 5 on question number 1, then he loves food enough for it to be a pleasurable experience, and he could use it to soothe himself. In this situation, make sure that you do not use food to soothe your child's emotions. It is okay for children to *like* food and treats, but it is detrimental for them to *need* it to soothe their emotions.

Spending time with your child is essential, and going for ice cream together is perfectly fine as long as you don't always use food to do so. As long as you are showing your love in other ways and telling your child you love her often, she won't connect food to being the only way to feel loved.

Have you heard the saying "Eat to live or live to eat"? Some of us cannot wait for our next meal or to try a new restaurant. Our lives are centered on one gastronomic experience after another; we *live to eat*. "Eat to live" folks eat because they need to for survival. They may or may not enjoy their meal, but they certainly are not thinking about or planning for the next eating experience until it happens again.

Be careful when children are in the "live to eat" camp, and avoid using food to soothe their emotions. Question #1 addresses these characteristics. Teach your child how to use other methods to feel better when he is sad, frustrated, or angry, especially if he scored a 4 or 5 on the scale. Have your child try exercising, playing, drawing, painting, listening to music, and talking with a friend; these are all great examples of ways to address emotions without covering feelings with food.

One last note: Never underestimate the power of saying "I love you" to your children, no matter how old they are. Everyone wants to know they are loved and that they matter. To lessen your children's need to reach to food for validation, remind them that you love them when they need it most, when they are acting out and pushing you away the hardest.

CHAPTER 3

Establish Food Rules at the Table

You have just served a meal to your family and now is
the time when the fur starts to fly with your picky eater.
You hold your breath—yes, you do—hoping everyone
will eat the food you prepared, that no one will
yell "Yuck!" and ruin the entire dinner, and you
keep your fingers crossed that your picky eater
does not ask you to cook another meal because
she does not want the one you just served.

If a child never has to face consequences for not eating the healthy food he needs, why would he eat healthy food?

In this chapter, you will learn how to manage the tricks and downright manipulative techniques picky eaters use with great success. Always remember that you are the one in charge and that you can handle anything that is thrown at you, even if you do not feel like that's the case at the moment. Keep a smile on your face and a calm tone, even if you feel like screaming and running from the room.

You will not be able to turn around a picky eater unless you have a set of food rules and subsequent consequences at home. I am so sure about this because there are no other social behaviors that our children "naturally" acquire without parents setting expectations and following through with consequences when those expectations are not met. Think about how you set a bedtime for your child or taught him to say "Please" and "Thank you," play nicely with friends, or clean up his room. If a child never has to face consequences for not eating the healthy food he needs, why would he eat healthy food? Would you if you didn't know the consequences of following an unhealthy diet? Probably not.

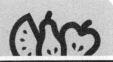

START WITH SUBTLETY

I do not recommend starting this program by announcing, "Things are going to change around here! Now I'm the boss at the table." If you want to start a war at home, this statement or attitude would certainly accomplish that. Instead, use subtleness in your approach and patience and consistency as your tools. In this chapter, you will learn how to do this while setting up food goals and consequences for your family.

You will now learn how to create and enforce rules and consequences for healthy eating. You will be able to distinguish between punishment and consequences, which rests in the way you enforce the rules. By setting up rules and following through with consequences over and over again, your picky eater will finally learn that she needs to eat the healthy stuff before she can have an unhealthy treat.

How to Set Up Rules and Consequences

Initially, you may be uncomfortable about setting rules around food, especially if you are an indulgent parent or have been instructed to back off at the table. I would encourage you to think about how effective rules and consequences are in establishing so many behaviors you desire in your child—wearing a helmet or sharing, for example. Why would this longstanding, tried-and-true discipline method not work in the realm of food?

It is time for you to set up a feeding method that works for your children—one that takes into account both your and your child's personality. To be most effective in developing rules in your household, there are certain essential elements, detailed in the following list, that will help you to succeed.

NOTE: As you take in the lessons throughout this book, I encourage you to use your inner guidance when working with your picky eater. Listening to what feels right to you and what doesn't is essential because, at the end of the day, no one knows your child better than you do.

1. Center yourself first.

Before you sit down for a meal, take your child grocery shopping, or even show her how to cook, make sure that you are centered. I am not asking you to remove all the stress in your life, but I am asking that you take a few deep breaths, turn off your phone and your internal multitasker, and focus on your child for the next few minutes. You are setting yourself up for disaster if you are pressed for time or going over your work project in your head while you are eating with your child or teaching her how to shop.

Try this centering exercise anywhere and anytime you need to calm down—no one will know that you are doing it. Take a minute to firmly plant your feet on the ground and take three long, deep breaths. Do not rush, but feel your incoming breath calming you. As you exhale, imagine your stress releasing through your out-breath. Those three deep, slow breaths will reset you.

2. Get your spouse on board.

Nothing is more confusing to children than when dad says one thing and mom says another. I could write an entire book dedicated to the issue of spouses and food. I have spoken to many wives who blame their husbands for sabotaging their efforts to serve their children a healthy diet. They talk about all the work they do to buy and prepare healthy food only to have their husband bring home ice cream or chips. I have also spoken to husbands who think their wives are over the top with concern. (Sometimes the wives are the unhealthy feeders, but that situation has been rare in my practice.)

Your chance of success with your picky eater is so much greater if you and your spouse are on the same page.

If this is the case in your household, I suggest that you read "The Life of Bryan" (see page 16) to your spouse, or better yet, have him or her read this book with you. After your spouse has more information on picky eaters, sit down when the two of you have time to connect. Allow each other to speak freely, without interruption, about your concerns with your child's diet. Your chance of success with your picky eater is so much greater if you and your spouse are on the same page. I have also covered the topic of spousal teamwork in *Beat Sugar Addiction Now! for Kids*; there is an entire section devoted to this topic, plus a homework assignment that helps to get your spouse on board.

If no amount of convincing can get your spouse to enforce the rules, make a deal that he or she will at least not purchase or feed your children unhealthy food while you are establishing the rules. Once your spouse sees how much easier mealtime becomes, he or she may very well join you in your efforts.

3. Recognize when to tighten or loosen the reins.

Understanding the issue of control is essential when bringing up children—not just when dealing with food and the picky eater. It takes us eighteen years (or more!) to prepare our children to go out into the world and make their own decisions. That is a long time. During this period, we start off with total control and slowly and with caution, pass some of that control to our children when they have demonstrated that they can handle it. The same process occurs when feeding your children.

You definitely want to give your children a sense of control when they are young, but make that control be their decision between two healthy options: Do you want milk or water with lunch? Would you like crackers and cheese or yogurt for a snack? A young child, especially one younger than three or four, does not have the cognitive ability to differentiate between a healthy choice and an unhealthy choice. Many older children and even some adults who have no understanding of the benefits and consequences of their food choices cannot make that decision well enough either.

As your children get older and begin to understand why making healthy eating choices is so important, you can hand them a little bit more control. But age is not the only indicator of when you should pass along more control. Two more factors are important: your children's understanding of what they need to eat and why they need to eat it, plus their ability to show you over time that they can make the right decision. You know how to do this, as you use this technique in dozens of other situations: can your children walk to the end of the block, can they ride their bike out of your sight, and so on? As they show you time and time again that they can make healthy choices, you can let up on the reins.

4. Be prepared by prepping your pantry.

Before you embark on rule setting, make sure your kitchen is stocked with healthy options. The worst thing that you can do is to tell your child he needs to eat his fruit first before he can have a cookie, and then have no fresh produce on hand. Getting the items on the following list is a good place to start:

- Fresh fruit

- Fresh vegetables, cut into sticks

- Healthy dips such as hummus

- Cheese

- Whole-grain crackers

- Low-fat yogurt

- Eggs

- Nuts (if no allergies are present)

Now that you know what kinds of foods you should have on hand, get rid of the junk food hanging around—empty your house, car, purse, and wherever else. I am not asking you to throw food away but to just stop buying soda, juice boxes, flavored drinks, candy, and gummy fruit snacks. Keep one or two treat options on hand for the week but no more—they will just be too tempting for everyone.

Six Simple and Effective Food Rules to Live By

You are now ready to learn the essential rules for turning around a picky eater. But these rules apply to all children, picky eaters or not. To be successful, you also need to lead by example so make sure you practice these rules and that your entire family knows that they need to follow them, including you.

1. Eat then treat.

The most essential piece of information that this generation of children needs to survive and thrive is to know the difference between healthy and unhealthy food. They have to face a world full of junk food at every turn, and they need to learn how to navigate through it. Our job as parents begins with teaching them to look upon these foods as unhealthy, junk, treats, or whatever term you want to use that gets the message across that these foods will not lead to health, longevity, reaching their potential, or optimal performance. To put it in kid-speak, they will not grow up big and strong if they eat too much unhealthy food and drink too many unhealthy beverages.

The most essential piece of information that this generation of children needs to survive and thrive is to know the difference between healthy and unhealthy food.

As with all other behaviors, like napping and using good manners, children need to be taught how to eat healthfully, each and every day. The "eat then treat" rule—of not getting the unhealthy stuff until they have eaten the healthy food—should be enforced at snack and mealtimes. Below are some examples of "eat then treat":

- No dessert until the meal is eaten

- No treat at snack time until a fruit or veggie is eaten

- No treats at all if enough healthy food was not eaten that day

When enforcing this rule, do so in an encouraging manner and not a threatening one. Saying "You are not getting ice cream until you eat your carrots!" in a negative tone or a raised voice is different than a matter-of-fact comment such as, "Oh, I see you haven't eaten your carrots. We are having ice cream for dessert. You can have some once you eat your carrots. The choice is yours." The first example makes you the boss while the second puts control into your child's hands.

The trick to setting rules is to leave your children with the impression that they are the ones in charge. Children need to know that they have some control over the food they eat, but the truth is they are too young to really understand how to make healthy selections. As your children grow, you will give more control to them once you see that they understand *how* to eat healthfully and that they will *choose* to eat healthfully when on their own most of the time.

I do not want you to think that I am promoting a treat with each meal or snack. On the contrary, if you look at the expendable calories your children have each day (see Appendix B: Daily Serving Guide for Children), it adds up to about one treat. What I am saying is that if you choose to give your children one treat a day, hold off giving it to them until they eat enough healthy food first. For some children, other foods or beverages can serve as the incentive: *Drinkers* (who fall under the Taster eating personalities), for example, need to eat their meal before getting their beverage.

Annoyance over trying a new food is okay; fear is not.

The "eat then treat" technique is different from using food as a reward; it is in fact just a consequence of healthy eating. Children's stomachs need to fill up on the required food and drink seen in the table in Appendix B (Daily Serving Guide for Children) before filling up on empty calories. Having said that, research suggests that "rewarding" children with one food when they eat another causes them to like the rewarded food more than if it wasn't used in this way. Do your children like cookies because they taste great, or do they love cookies because they know they cannot have them all the time? I suspect it mostly has to do with great taste, but I also realize the lure of forbidden fruit—er, candy.

Consequences: The consequences of "eat then treat" are simple: If your child does not eat his healthy dinner or the healthy part of his snack first, he does do not get his treat. Period. This is the quickest way to turn around a picky eater.

2. Establish the one-bite rule.

The first time a child tastes a new food, she may not like it because the taste or texture is foreign or it reminds her of something else that she does not like (e.g., "I didn't like orange carrots so I am not going to like orange sweet potatoes."). Encouraging a child to take the first bite of a new food is essential in order to have it move onto the list of foods he will eat. Your child's diet will not be varied—and a varied diet is the most nutritious diet there is—unless you establish this rule at home.

Expect younger children, and some older children, to make a face when they try a new food. Here is the key: DO NOT REACT. Remain calm and matter-of-fact. Your children will look to see whether they are going to get a reaction out of you. Children can determine which adult in their life they can manipulate at the dinner table faster than the speed of the Internet. If you look at them with eyes that say "Please, oh please, like this food," you will most likely get the opposite reaction from them. If they know that you will leave the new food off the menu after one displeased look or reaction, they will use that reaction each and every time to get out of eating the stuff they do not want to eat.

When you first introduce a new food to your child, let her know that she just has to take one bite that she can spit out if she does not like it. Spitting out is only allowed on the first introduction to a new food. If your child does not have an intense reaction like gaging or throwing up after the first exposure, chances are it is a food that you can continue to encourage. Next time, she has to try two bites, then three, and so on until she has eaten an appropriate serving of the new food.

For a child who is extremely resistant to trying new foods, consider using a system that gives the child a sticker or a certain amount of points that may earn him quality time with you or extra playtime with his friends, each time he reaches his goal: one bite, two bites, etc. You may also need to implement the touch-smell-lick approach for children who are very fearful of new foods. First, have your child touch the new food, even play with it. Then have him smell it, and if he is comfortable with it, have him lick it before you ask him to take a bite.

Consequences: How much do you push your child to take a bite of a new food? This is the number one question I get from most parents of picky eaters. The answer: This is where your expertise in your children is essential. You know your children better than anyone else. You know whether they are being stubborn and trying to control a situation, and you know when they are truly upset. Children will experience some distress when trying a new food because they simply do not want to try the new food. Some children, however, get so emotional over a bite of a new food that they shake, scream, or move their head back and forth violently. All of these expressions are signs that the situation is too much for your child. Annoyance over trying a new food is okay; fear is not.

If you pair fear with a food, the results can be quite drastic. Do you remember vomiting after eating a certain food when you came down with the stomach flu as a child? I bet that to this day there is a food that you cannot go near because you have such a negative memory of it. You have literally created a taste aversion to that food: You paired the sick feeling with the food, and that is hard to undo.

The same thing happens if you push a child so far that fear is introduced when they taste the new food. If that happens, the child will have a taste aversion to that food, and to make matters worse, the child will often associate that food with others like it. For instance, if a child had to eat her green beans and she was afraid of eating them, she may want to avoid all green vegetables because they elicit fear, too.

Children can determine which adult in their life they can manipulate at the dinner table faster than the speed of the Internet.

Do not force them to overeat, but let children know that food is a precious resource and as such it should not be discarded so readily.

3. Serve a fruit or veggie with every meal and snack.

For children to have the full complement of all the building blocks they need to create their body, construct strong bones, establish strong neural connections, develop a strong immune system, and so on, they need to eat lots of fruits and vegetables— at least two whole fruits and three vegetables a day. The special nutrients in these foods are called phytonutrients, and they provide superpowers for your children.

To include the required amount of fruits and vegetables in a child's diet, a child practically needs to eat one or the other at every meal and snack. If they do not need to eat a snack, then they need to eat both a fruit and vegetable with their meals. Most children do not see a vegetable until at least lunchtime, and that means that to get their three servings a day, they need one serving of vegetables at lunch, one for snack, and one for dinner. The two fruit servings are usually easier to get into a child's daily routine—you can serve fruit at breakfast and snack time.

Many children prefer fruit to vegetables, and at lunch, they are more likely to eat their fruit but leave the vegetable off the tray or out of the lunchbox. Get children into the habit of having a vegetable with lunch because it is an unreasonable expectation to think they will eat three servings of vegetables at dinner. Do not resort to vegetable juices (especially those mixed with fruit juice)—they do not count as a vegetable serving in my book.

Consequences: If children do not eat their two servings of whole fruit and three servings of vegetables per day, they do not get any processed treats. Those include cookies, cakes, puddings, ice cream, and other obvious choices, as well as chips and the less obvious non-whole-grain crackers (especially those in animal shapes), gummy fruit treats (these do not count as a fruit), breakfast bars, and other granola bars. Implement the "eat then treat rule" to get children used to the taste of vegetables and whole fruit.

4. Limit food waste.

The amount of food waste in the United States is out of control: We produce 34 million tons of it a year, enough to feed everyone in America with leftovers. Some of us grew up hearing the admonishment "Eat your dinner because there are starving children in Africa." Parents used this common technique in the past to get their children to eat everything on their plate, but often this convinced children to eat beyond fullness, which is never a good idea.

The anti-clean-your-plate club actually did great work in stopping the practice of forcing children to eat everything on their plate. Although I am happy that parents now know not to force their children to clean their plate, I am discouraged by what I see as a side effect of this teaching: Many children today have no regard for food, and as such, they throw away a lot of it out without a second thought. If you doubt this, visit a school cafeteria. You will be shocked by how much food is thrown away on a typical day. In fact, about 12 percent of food served in the National School lunch program in 2002 was thrown away. The cost of this wastefulness is a whopping $600 million a year.

I often see picky eaters sit down to a meal, take one or two bites, and leave the table with no awareness that they are wasting food. Within 10 to 20 minutes, they all come back asking for a snack. If parents give in—as they usually do—they end up feeding their children enough snacks to make up for the calories their children should have gotten from their meal. I do think that a happy medium can be met: Do not force them to overeat, but let children know that food is a precious resource and as such it should not be discarded so readily.

Learning to value food comes from you, and it starts by letting your children know that what is not eaten at mealtime will be served again afterward when they are hungry. The next time your picky eater takes a couple of bites, announces he is full, and leaves the table, say, "If you are full you may be excused, but know that when you are hungry again, your meal will be your only option," or when he comes back asking for a snack, say "Snacks are not an option until you have eaten your meal." Your children learn to be wasteful from you, so if you throw away their food without any consequences, you are sending the message that you do not value food either.

To practice this rule most effectively, make sure that you have a good understanding of what a serving size is for your child. I cover appropriate serving sizes in the next chapter, and you can find the amount of food that your child needs to consume in a day in Appendix B. If you know, for example, that a two-year-old can be expected to eat 2 tablespoons of vegetables, a four-year-old ¼ cup, and a ten-year-old ½ cup, then you will be able to set reasonable expectations at the table. Setting the limit-food-waste rule lets children know that you expect them to eat what is served. If the serving size was appropriate and they are not able to finish what is on their plate, that is fine. Just let them know that the next time they are hungry they will be offered the food left on their plate.

If your children do not want to eat the meal that was prepared for them, ask them to sit at the table while everyone else eats.

Consequences: The next time your picky eater sits down to a meal and takes one or two bites and pushes her plate away, remain calm. Ask your child whether she is full. If she says yes, let her know that the next time she is hungry she will be served her meal again. If she is still hungry, tell her she needs to eat what is served because that is her only choice: Take it or leave it. Either way, your picky eater is sure to be put off the first time you call her bluff. Just remain firm with a smile on your face and repeat that this is the meal and do not offer after-dinner snacks or dessert until she has eaten her meal.

5. Serve only one dinner.

You made chicken and rice and your children want hot dogs. What do you do? If you are the mom of the *Short Order Diner* (chapter 6), you have probably thrown a hot dog into the pot with annoyance and served it. You thought that providing a meal your children would eat was better than them not eating at all. Now you know better. You realize that liking a food is something that your children need to learn, and they won't learn to like a new food if they never have to eat it.

A practical reason for installing the "one dinner" rule is that being a short order chef does not work for anyone's busy lifestyle, especially if you have multiple kids sitting down to one meal. Serving several different meals does not teach children to eat what is served to them, either.

For those of you who have children who ask for separate meals, before you prepare the family dinner, it is essential that you get their input—for example, ask, "What vegetable you would prefer—peas or broccoli?" Give each child a turn to pick the theme or main dish for dinner on one night of the week. Knowing that they have a say in what is being served on some nights of the week helps to get them on board for those nights when they didn't have any input. Dinner provides a great opportunity to try new foods and tastes.

Consequences: If your children do not want to eat the meal that was prepared for them, ask them to sit at the table while everyone else eats. If they become unruly, excuse them to go to their room in a nonchalant way. Do not permit them to engage in electronics or any other play. This is essentially like a time-out. When everyone is done with dinner, they may come out of their room. When they are hungry, offer them the dinner that you prepared.

Many parents have an opt-out option for when their child does not like dinner. I do not think this is a good idea because it basically enables your picky eater to eat only a few select foods. If the opt-out option is healthy and easy to throw together, such as a plate of cut-up veggies and dip, go for it, but more than likely it looks something like this: a peanut butter and jelly sandwich, mac 'n' cheese, microwavable pizza snacks, and other quick-and-easy processed options.

6. No "yuck" is allowed at the table.

Most of us with more than one child have experienced the frustration of serving a great meal only to have it ruined by one little word that has a major impact. Imagine (or remember back to when) you have spent thirty minutes or more making a healthy meal only to have it completely ruined when one of your little darlings takes a bite and yells "Yuck!" Everyone else under the age of eighteen immediately drops their fork, even if they were enjoying their meal.

Let your children know that the next time they yell "yuck" at the table, they will be immediately excused and given a time-out in their room. Follow the same process you would with a regular time-out: one minute maximum for each year of age (maximum of 10 minutes) or until they have calmed down enough and are ready to return. Explain to your children that saying "yuck" about the meal you've made is like when they have just spent the afternoon making a huge sandcastle and excitedly ask you to come over and see it, but before you get there, their sibling destroys it. Ask them how they would feel. Let them know that when you create a dinner for them, you do not like it being destroyed by that one little word either.

Teach your children that they can express themselves by saying "This is not my favorite" or "I would rather have chicken instead" or some other subtle and respectful way of saying they don't like what you served them. Let it end there. After one of my sons lets me know that he does not like what I just served for dinner, I let him know "You may not like it; you just need to eat it" or "You may not like it, but it likes you." Only use these examples or encourage your children to eat those foods that are in the "I don't love it but I don't hate it" category and do not push any food in the "I really hate it" realm. I do not let them use the words "I don't like" to get out of having to eat any food they do not want to eat, but I also never, ever make them eat something they really despise.

Consequences: Whenever "yuck" is heard at the table, give your child a time-out. Leave his food on the table and when his time-out is over, he may rejoin the family. Don't make the time-out more than five or ten minutes, though—you do not want his dinner to get too cold. When your child returns to the table, do not make a big deal over his outburst or fuss over him. Just tell them once, "We do not say yuck at the table," and then continue on with your meal. Your child's siblings will be watching you for a reaction, and you do not want to give your picky eater extra attention for this rude behavior.

Five Steps for Laying Down the Law

Here are five steps you can use for implementing the six food rules and following through with their consequences. These steps will help you on your way to creating a peaceful mealtime.

Step 1: Inform your children.

Once you have reviewed the rules in this chapter, choose a time when no one is in a rush and call a family meeting. Start by describing the rules that will be established in your home regarding food and behavior at the table and in general. Follow up with what the consequences will be for not following the rules.

Explain to your children that the food rules are in place for their health, so that they can reach their potential. Do not expect them to like the rules or to jump on board with enthusiasm right away. What you most likely will get instead is resistance and fear. They will react as if you said you would be taking away their favorite toy. When they react, it is best not to respond but to instead take a deep breath and validate their feelings. Try saying, "I understand that you do not like these rules and they make you angry. These rules are going to help all of us eat a healthy diet, which is important for making us healthy and strong."

Children do not like change, especially if it means that they do not get their way. Focus on the positive and assure them that there will be lots of great tasty food they will end up loving and that all of you will be spending more time together as a family.

Step 2: Implement one rule at a time.

No one likes it when a bunch of rules are dumped on them at once. When you start to implement food rules in your household, begin by setting realistic expectations. If you currently let your child have free reign when it comes to food, transition them to the new way of doing things by selecting one rule to focus on at a time.

To start, choose the rule that you feel would make the most positive change in your child's eating habits or one that seems easy so that you get your child on board quickly. The decision as to which rule to start with is up to you and your family situation at the moment. You may even consider getting your children's input on which rule to start with, as that would add a degree of buy-in from them.

Once your children have learned one rule, move on to the next one. Do not expect your children to embrace and enjoy a rule before moving on to the next one, however. Before moving forward, you want the battle to be over, but there may still be complaints now and again. Continue implementing rule-by-rule until you have taught your children what you expect from them at the table.

Children do not like change, especially if it means that they do not get their way.

Step 3: Display the rules.

I encourage you to make a list of the food rules that everyone, including adults, must follow. Have your child create a nice design on a small poster board and write the rules on it for everyone to see. If you have more than one child, everyone can add his or her artwork to the rule list. There is also a pullout list of the rules in Appendix A. Post the rules where your family usually eats their meals. You many need one poster in the kitchen and one in the dining room.

The next time your children ask whether they need to eat their vegetables, point to the rule list, your external reminder and prop.

Step 4: Enforce the rules.

Enforcing the rules and making sure your child follows them is where current recommendations fall short. It is why many of us pull our hair out with frustration day in and day out. The reason for this is that a child's unique eating personality is not taken into account when we are guided in getting children to eat healthfully.

The most popular method, which instructs us to put food in front of our children and let them decide what they want to eat, works for very few children, especially when processed food is in the mix. It will not work for the *Player*, who is so distracted and has a hard time staying seated at the table, or the *Junk-Food Junkie*, who just wants sweet treats. In section 2 of this book, you will discover how to individualize your follow-through and enforcement of the rules for every eating personality and character.

In general, remain calm throughout the meal, even if it means you need to remove yourself from the table for a few minutes. We all get frustrated when dealing with a picky eater. Sometimes it is all I can do to keep my cool when my son takes a very long time to finish his meal. In times like these, I remind myself that it won't be like this forever. If my son takes forever to eat his meal, I give him two choices: He can stay at the table as long as he is eating or he can go to his room until he is hungry again. As soon as emotions escalate at the table, I know that I have lost my opportunity for success. When a mealtime turns into a war, it cannot be a learning environment.

After the consequence is over, do not draw undue attention or continue to discuss the rule breaking. Keep any reprimand short and simple because most children tune out after a few sentences: "We do not say yuck; it ruins the meal for everyone." Try to focus on the positive more than the negative. Make a big deal the next time you see your picky eater doing something right: "Great job eating your peas!" or "What a fabulous job you did eating your chicken! You are sure to grow up big and strong."

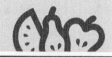

PUNISHMENT VERSUS RULES AND CONSEQUENCES

Most likely you already know how to enforce rules and consequences in your house if your child is polite, goes to bed at a reasonable hour, and plays outside most days of the week. When learning how to set up expectations around food, think about how you would get your children to do their homework when they would rather play with their toys or electronics. Would you sit them down to explain why they needed to do their homework? You probably would in the beginning, but you wouldn't use information as your only tactic.

More than likely you would pull out other strategies to get them to do what they needed to do. You might tell them "it is time to do your homework." You'd remind them again, and then, if you are still not being heard, you'd amp it up a bit: "If you do not do your homework, there is going to be no TV watching tonight," or some other consequence along the lines of "If this is not done, then you do not get that."

Think of processed food like the toy or video game and the healthy food as the homework. Most children prefer the toy to the homework; in fact, they would rather play with the toy all day and never get to the homework. Unless they had to do their homework, they would not. Isn't the same thing happening at the dinner table? If a child does not "have to" eat the healthy stuff, will he? In my experience, he will not.

No screaming or physical punishment is ever needed; instead, use explanations and time-outs. If you find that you are losing your patience, then take a time-out yourself. Here are some "never-evers" regarding food with children:

- Never use physical or undue emotional force to make your child eat a bite of food.

- Never force your child to finish a meal.

- Stop what you are doing if your child gets emotionally upset or cries.

- Stop what you are doing if your child gags or vomits.

- Never hit your child for not eating what you want her to; physical force is never constructive or permitted.

- Do not raise your voice at the table.

- Do not threaten your child if he does not eat.

Step 5: Be consistent when it comes to food rules.

Being consistent about following the rules and invoking consequences is so essential that you should not start implementing the rules unless you are ready to stick to them. The reason for this is that children are really good at knowing which buttons to push and which parent is the softy, and they will use all their charm and manipulative skills to break the rules and dodge the consequences. You need to be ready for this, to know that your child will push your guilt button sooner than you can say "Broccoli, anyone?"

Children are smarter than you think, and they will do what they are genetically programmed to do: survive. Their genetic survival instinct to eat and preference for tasty processed foods creates children who are super-strong-willed about getting their way around food and who do not back down easily. You have probably heard children scream and cry that they were starving. When you hear this, your parenting instinct to keep your child alive kicks in, and more times than not, you will hand them the bag of chips that was the focus of the fuss in the first place.

Now that you understand all of this—that no one is to blame and both parent and child are following instinctual impulses—it is time to use your cognition. The next time this scene unfolds—and it will, trust me—take a breath, assess the situation (is my child starving?), and calmly say, "No, you may not have that bag of chips. We are going home for dinner," or "No, you cannot have that bag of chips, but here is an apple instead." If they are truly hungry, the apple will be eaten; if not, starvation wasn't happening—a craving was. Your job as a parent is to distinguish between the two. Truly hungry children without physical or mental disorders will usually eat a fruit or vegetable, but children who are craving sweets and salt will pass.

Once you have started setting up the rules and following through with the consequences, stick with the game plan 100 percent. If you let the rules or consequences slip, especially in the beginning, you are essentially sending a mixed message, which confuses children. Also, as soon as you start to show any wiggle room, your children will come barging in.

I realize that always enforcing the rules may seem overwhelming and that you may feel that you are being too strict, especially if you are an indulgent parent. It is during these times, however, that you need to remind yourself that this period of "strict rules" will not last forever and that you are doing this for your children's best interests. In the long run, everyone will have an easier time because you have stuck with the rules.

Once rules are firmly established, you can back off slightly just as you would with any other rule you set for your child. Take bedtime as an example. How often do you let your children stay up past their bedtime? If you do it too often, you will need to spend a period of time resetting expectations. You already know how to do this; I am just inviting you to use the same methods that work for you in many other areas of your children's lives and bring them into the realm of food.

CHAPTER 4

How to Set the Stage for a Pleasant Meal

The following scene is one that plays out on most nights of the week during mealtime: children arguing, dogs running around, phones ringing or texts flying back and forth, and your children leaving the table before they have had enough to eat. No one, especially a picky eater, can eat in this type of frenzied environment. Mealtime should be a time in our busy day when everyone connects and nourishes themselves with food and time together. Bringing back family meals is one of the ways to turn around your picky eater.

Only a truly hungry child will eat his or her meal.

Who wants to come to dinner when it is a stressful affair? No one I know. The good news is that mealtimes don't have to be stressful in your house no matter how busy your schedule is. You can set the stage so your family's physical and emotional environment is one that encourages peace, fun, connection, and of course, healthy eating.

In addition to reducing stress around mealtime, it is important that your picky eater come to the table hungry! One of the most essential pieces of information that you will learn in this book is that only a truly hungry child will eat his or her meal. If you let your children snack two hours before a meal, you cannot expect them to eat enough of their meal. When children do not eat their meals and instead rely on snacks and dessert to fill up, they will not get all the nutrients their growing bodies need.

Although most of the focus with picky eaters has been on how well they meet their nutritional requirements, there is another equally important, nourishing element of mealtime. When people gather to eat a meal, they bond and make connections, which is also essential for children's well-being. Every society uses food as an opportunity to take a break from the busy day and enjoy one another's company.

This chapter will introduce four table rules and four essential tips to prevent chaos from occurring at your dinner table. Think of mealtime as a performance, and the way you prepare the environment is the stage you set. Limiting distractions and making the environment pleasant will dramatically increase your chances of having a great meal. Begin the process of stopping mealtime chaos and determine your family's current eating environment by answering the following questions.

What Does Mealtime Look Like at Your Home?

1 How do you usually act at the table?

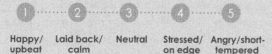

| Happy/upbeat | Laid back/calm | Neutral | Stressed/on edge | Angry/short-tempered |

2 How does your spouse act at the table?

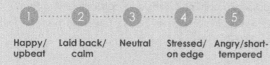

| Happy/upbeat | Laid back/calm | Neutral | Stressed/on edge | Angry/short-tempered |

3 On the scale below, which description best fits your child's energy level at the table?

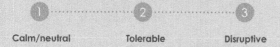

Calm/neutral   Tolerable   Disruptive

4 Are you usually rushed for time during meals?

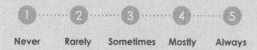

Never   Rarely   Sometimes   Mostly   Always

5 How often is someone yelling or arguing at the table during mealtime?

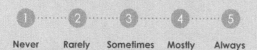

Never   Rarely   Sometimes   Mostly   Always

6 Do you usually have the TV, radio, or other electronics going while eating meals?

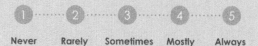

Never   Rarely   Sometimes   Mostly   Always

7 If you have pets, do they come to the table at mealtime and interact with your children?

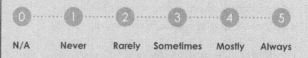

N/A   Never   Rarely   Sometimes   Mostly   Always

8 Do you usually eat at a table (instead of on the living room couch or chairs, in a bedroom, etc.)?

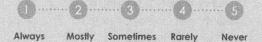

Always   Mostly   Sometimes   Rarely   Never

9 How often do you eat together as a family?

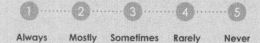

Always   Mostly   Sometimes   Rarely   Never

10 How many times does someone from your family get up from the table during mealtime?

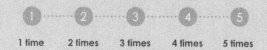

1 time   2 times   3 times   4 times   5 times

Add up your score and determine where you fall on the mealtime-stress-o-meter:

39 to 48: Yikes! Time for a mealtime overhaul.

Mealtime in your household is full of distractions and chaos. It is not healthy to pair the stress that comes from all the chaos with the act of eating. In this type of environment, people cannot hear their inner cues: The chaos overrides any messages their stomachs are giving them to stop or continue eating. Your child will either undereat or overeat depending on his or her personality—in other words, do your children shut down or become overexcited when their physical and emotional environments are frantic? Either way, this is not the environment in which you should sit down to dinner—much less the type of environment in which you can successfully turn around a picky eater.

25 to 38: On the edge of chaos.

Your score indicates that your family is in the middle ground between chaos and peace at mealtime. Depending on everyone's personality or how his or her day went, the stress at the table may be too overwhelming to allow your family to focus on healthy eating. Even if the frenzy does not seem to bother everyone on the outside, the stress is impossible to ignore and some people internalize it instead. There is room for improvement at your dinner table.

9 to 24: Great environment for eating.

You are doing a great job in providing a calm and focused eating environment for your family. Keep up the great work making sure that external stimuli is kept out of your dining room or kitchen while your family sits down together to share a meal. Keep reading to find out why it is so important to continue doing what you are doing and make sure you are mirroring healthy eating habits as well as serving appropriate portions to your children.

Four Table Rules to Prevent Mealtime Chaos and Encourage Family Connection

Now that you know where you stand regarding mealtime chaos, you can begin to create a pleasant eating environment by using the following table rules.

Table Rule #1: Everyone has a job to do at mealtime.

Everyone in your family needs to become involved in getting a meal to the table. This means that your children need to help out in the kitchen, dining room, grocery store, and garden, if you have one. Your children can select one area to focus on each week, because being involved in all aspects at once can be too overwhelming, especially for younger children.

Your ultimate goal, however, is to teach your children enough so that when they are teenagers and going off to college, trade school, or elsewhere, they will be able to create a meal from start to finish. Seventeen and eighteen-year olds should be able to accomplish this task with practice: have your teen cook one meal every week. In the meantime, give a weekly chore to the younger or older child who has never been involved in the making of a meal before. See specific suggestions in the sidebar "How Kids Can Help Plan, Pick, Prep, and Cook."

HOW KIDS CAN HELP PLAN, PICK, PREP, AND COOK

Here are specific ways that you can get your children, no matter their age, involved in getting a meal on the table. Your children can:

Set the table and clean up afterward. Even the youngest of children can put a spoon and napkins on the table; the older child can place knives, forks, and beverages. To add an element of fun, have your child create a theme for the table by picking certain placemats or decorations. For cleanup, everyone's least favorite job, have your child put on an apron and pretend he is a waiter and teach him to collect plates the "official" way, from the right.

Help shop for groceries. Create a grocery list before you step into a supermarket and give your child the job of finding items on that list. If you dread shopping with your picky eater, let her choose one treat for the week. When your child is helping you shop and asks for something that is not on the list, first tell her she cannot have it but that she can pick out her one treat. If she keeps asking or whining or escalates to screaming, take away her privilege of getting her treat. You will not have to do this more than once or twice before your picky eater learns to behave.

Help garden. *Gardening* in this context is meant very loosely. It can include picking produce from the garden when it is ripe, picking herbs from pots on the windowsill, participating in a community garden, or trying to grow a bean seed in a paper cup on your windowsill. No matter where you live, try to introduce the experience of growing a plant from seed to your children.

The awareness that something as small as a seed can grow into something bigger and edible is an essential element of understanding that children need to learn what food is and is not. It is also an opportunity for you to promote eating fresh produce: When your children see that a plant needs sunlight and water to grow, they learn that they also need sunlight and water to grow. During the winter months, have your children select fresh produce from the store and your refrigerator.

Help in the kitchen. Have your children wash and cut up produce, measure and stir, or follow a recipe—it all depends on their age and skill level. Picky eaters need to become familiar with the food they are going to be asked to eat, so what better way than to have them wash, peel, and use it in a recipe? If they have participated in the creation of the meal, their chances of trying a new food increases because it is not so new to them anymore.

Think of the grocery store, kitchen, garden, and dining room table as nutrition classrooms. The soil, store, sink, countertop, and table are where your child learns how food grows, how to prepare it, how to select the healthiest options, and how to eat it. All these areas help your children learn from an experiential perspective, which solidifies what

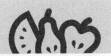

they are also learning in school and at the doctor's office. It is one thing to tell children to eat healthfully; it is entirely another to show them how.

While you are cooking, shopping, planting, and eating with your children, share with them facts about healthy eating along with your personal experiences. Show them how you used to make bread with your grandmother, for example, or create a dish from your heritage. All of these acts weave food into the tapestry of who your children are, and it certainly beats repeating the same old information: eat your veggies. Food becomes part of your children's life in an intimate way when you make meals personal for your family.

Consequences: Create a list of your children's meal-related tasks and place it where they can see it so they can determine beforehand what is expected of them. Rotate these chores so each of your children has exposure to all the many facets of food. To be fair, all parents need to get involved in the preparation and cleaning up of a meal. (I am speaking mainly to the spouses—you know who you are.) If your children do not do their task, instill the same consequences for them that you would use when they do not complete their other chores, such as taking away a privilege or decreasing their weekly allowance.

Table Rule #2: Eat at the table.

Establishing this rule—that eating occurs only at the table—is important for focusing your picky eater. Can you imagine a kindergarten teacher having to chase her class around the school to teach them their ABCs?

Taking a break from the day and sitting down to a meal provides you with the opportunity to help your picky eater focus on and enjoy a well-balanced meal. Stopping what your children are doing and changing the scenery is like hitting a reset button: Now it is time to do something else—eat. It is also essential if you have children who would rather play than eat (see The *Player* on page 160). This eating personality has a hard time concentrating on the meal, instead preferring to be doing something else—anything else that doesn't require sitting still.

Start by dedicating a spot in your house that will serve as your dining room table. If you do have a dining room table that you save for special occasions, I suggest that you consider eating together as a family as the most special of occasions and use it often. Many families preserve their dining room for parties or use it as an office or storage space. If this describes your situation, start by removing all items that do not belong there and rediscover your table's purpose. If you do not have a dining room, a kitchen table will work just as well once you clear the table of items that do not belong there.

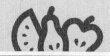

HOW TO GET EVERYONE TO THE TABLE

If you currently do not eat together as a family at the table, try these steps.

Step 1: To your current routine, add one dinner a week when everyone gathers for a meal. The more often you eat together as a family, the healthier your children's eating behavior will become. Research shows that families who eat together have young adults who eat more healthfully when they leave the house and eat on their own than those who do not.

Step 2: Continue to make eating together a priority until you either eat together on most nights of the week or you have reached your limit of eating together as a family. To bring everyone together, you need to decide as a family that being together at meals is your goal. Having said that, busy schedules are a reality in most households today; only you will be able to figure out how many times you can realistically eat as a family.

Step 3: If eating together does not seem to be a possibility or you can only manage to do so a couple times a week, try these strategies:

- If your children are so young that they cannot wait for daddy or mommy to come home to eat, let them eat their dinner earlier and save their snack for later while the adults eat.

- If sports keep you running late into the night, set aside weekend dinners as a time to get together. During the week, eat a snack together after the game or practice.

- Eat breakfast together as a family if dinners are never a possibility.

- For snack time, serve your picky eaters at the table, too. Sit down with them while they eat to encourage their cooperation. If they continue to grab snacks on the go, take the snacks away and sit them down at the table. If the grabbing gets out of hand, move their snacks from an easy-to-reach place to one where they do not have access to it.

- Do not serve a snack within two hours of mealtime. A hungry child will eat while a child who is semi-full or full on snacks will not. You will be surprised how effective this two-hour "no snacking" time is on their eating habits. Our society has gotten so out of control in terms of snacking that children often come to the table with no sense of hunger. Try it out and see how hunger is essential in turning around your picky eater. It may or may not be the complete answer, but it certainly is an important piece of the puzzle.

Consequences: If your child does not want to eat with everyone else, excuse him from the table without dinner. When he is hungry, he may return. If everyone is finished and he decides to eat, serve him dinner at the table. "I'm glad you decided to eat dinner. You must be hungry" is all you need to say. Your child will quickly learn that he needs to eat with the family or not at all. It may just take going to bed hungry one night to show him you mean business (don't do this if your child has diabetes or other issues). Serve him a big, healthy breakfast the next morning, and do not make a big deal of what happened last night beyond saying "You must be hungry, let's eat."

Eating in the living room, in front of the TV or computer, or on the couch is not conducive to focusing on your meal because eating becomes an afterthought instead of the centerpiece. In this case, eating is something you do while doing something else, like watching TV. This scattering of attention distracts the picky eater and everyone else.

When you're not focused on eating during mealtime, overeating is easy to do. You've probably had the experience of sitting down to watch TV or a movie and finishing a candy bar or bag of chips before you even realized that you were doing it. You look down in confusion and wonder where it went. This may sound like a good strategy for distracting a picky eater, but it needs to be used cautiously. Your goal is to focus your children so they can taste and feel and swallow their food without rushing, arguing, and fussing.

Food is not a pill to swallow quickly and get over with, although for many picky eaters this is exactly how it feels. If you give in to the quick fix of distraction all the time, you will actually promote picky eating, not reverse it. There may be moments where you need distraction to help your picky eater taste a new food, but after that, focus, not distraction, is the goal. You will learn more about this in section 2.

Table Rule #3: Electronics are not allowed at the table when eating.

If it requires a plug or battery, it remains off during mealtime, plain and simple. This means no phones or any other handheld entertainment devices. The television and radio are also tuned off. You want to teach picky eaters to settle down and decide what they want to eat, pay attention to their internal cues, focus on the taste of the food, and learn how to eat properly. This cannot be accomplished with the many distractions that electronics bring.

If your child has a hard time with her weight or eats lots of junky snack food, consider broadening your house rule to include no eating any time the television, computer, or other electronic device is on. A lot of mindless snacking on junk food occurs when children are zoned out in front of a screen. This rule also limits the impulse to grab a soda or cookie when a commercial for these items come on.

Show by example that a top priority for your family is for everyone to turn off the rest of the world and draw together as a family at least once a day. This means that no one, including you, brings a phone to the table. If your phone rings during mealtime, let voicemail pick it up. When you do this, you show your children how important they are to you and that family time is precious.

Because everyone has to eat, meals become the only time that a family has left in its busy day to bond and catch up on one another's activities. With this no-electronics rule, your children, including your picky eater, will get the message loud and clear that family is more important than anything else that may be going on in the world right now.

Consequences: If your child brings his phone or other handheld device to the table, take it away for the rest of the meal. If he gives you a hard time about this rule, then take the device away for the rest of the evening. Make a show of putting your phone away and not using it for the rest of the evening, too. Leading by example is the only way to set this rule effectively.

Table Rule #4: Whoever raises his or her voice leaves the table.

When everyone is rushed at mealtime, they tend to speak in loud voices to be heard above the chaos. Or the frantic energy proves to be too much for someone to take and they burst out yelling in frustration. No matter the reason, do no permit yelling at the table. Once you have set into place steps to create a calming environment, you will probably experience much less screaming at the table.

This rule, as with all others, applies to everyone at the table, including parents. Once the mood at dinner has escalated to a point where one or several family members are raising their voices or screaming, call a time-out. What that means is that you remove anyone raising his or her voice. If your child is the one getting out of hand, have him leave the table and go to his room (without electronics) to sit and calm down. Tell him that he may return when he can eat peacefully.

Mealtime also can be when everyone releases a bit of steam, especially after a long stressful day. If you have not connected with your child before dinnertime, do not be surprised to encounter some attitude and hostility sent your way during the meal. Children do not know how to say to you directly that they need more time with you. They usually speak with actions that seem the opposite of what they really want: They push you away in anger when they actually want you to spend more time with them. If you or your spouse can take ten minutes to play or bond with your children before dinner, you will allow them to blow off some steam and ultimately limit the chance for explosions at the table.

No one likes to eat in a stressful environment. It doesn't feel good, and it weaves strong negative emotions together with food. This is a perfect storm for creating an emotional eater. When you put together eating with yelling or anxiety from being a super-strict parent, you are teaching your child to turn to food for emotional comfort. Keep yelling and negative emotions out of your dining room as best you can.

Consequences: Whoever raises his or her voice gets a time-out. The rule of thumb is usually one minute per age, so a four-year-old would be on a time-out for four minutes. Limit an older child's time-out to five to ten minutes so that her dinner won't get so cold that she will no longer eat it. If she refuses to finish her meal, calmly tell her that if she is hungry before bedtime she can have her dinner again. Put her plate in the refrigerator and heat it up when she comes back for it later.

If you lose your cool at the table, give yourself a time out, too. Calm down in another room by taking some long deep breaths, punching a pillow, or listening to some soothing music. You do need to return to the table before everyone has finished eating. It is best not to be gone for more than five minutes because you don't want to teach your child that anyone can just escape from mealtime by yelling. When you get back to the table, continue to finish your dinner. If you feel an apology is in order, keep it brief and genuine: "I lost my cool. Mommy is sorry." The same advice holds true for your children—if they yell, they need to apologize to everyone as well.

When You Need Another Table Rule

Now is the time to add other table rules that you think are needed in your household. For example, some parents—such as friends of mine who have four boys!—don't allow burping or farting at the table. Feel free to add the table rules to your food rules list so that you put your expectations front and center.

Just make sure that you do not put too many rules up at once because it will overwhelm even the most easygoing child. As children begin to understand what is expected of them at the table, remove things from the lists of food and table rules that no longer are a problem but keep those items that your children need as reminders.

Four Essential Tips to Set the Stage for a Pleasant Meal

Implementing the table rules will be a lot easier with the help of the following four tips. Think of these four tips as the backdrop from which you present and reinforce the table rules. It may feel like acting at times because you will be smiling when you feel like screaming, remaining calm as you ask your child for the tenth time to stop leaving the table. And the Academy Award goes to . . . you.

Tip #1: Allow enough time to eat.

The quickest way to ruin a meal is to rush it. Every parent knows that children do not like to be rushed. How effective is yelling at your children to hurry and get dressed because you have an early work meeting or their bus is coming? Probably not much. Sometimes, in the heat of the moment, I think that children purposely dig in their feet and slow down when we need them to move quicker. They are actually just reacting to the stress and shutting down, and you'll probably receive the same response if you rush them to eat their meal.

Some of you think that you do not have all the time in the world, which is what it would take to sit there while your picky eater . . . well . . . picks. In our hurried day, when we finally are able to sit down to a meal and relax, we find ourselves getting stressed all over again because our picky eater eats so slowly or not at all. I am not asking you to allow an unreasonable amount of time for your children to pick at their meal, but that you set aside twenty to thirty minutes each night to allow for a leisurely meal and for your picky eater to finish it.

Twenty to thirty minutes is not a long time when you think about it, but it will seem like forever in the beginning, especially if your family rushes through its meal. If you do not believe me, look at the clock the next time your family sits down to eat—chances are most of your family members gobble and go in less than ten minutes.

It is hard for any of us after a long day to settle down and relax. We are still in a hyper, multitasking mode. You will need to train not only your picky eater but the rest of your family, including yourself, to eat in an unrushed, relaxing, and mindful way. At first, your family will probably finish meals quickly. Do not get up; instead, spend the rest of your twenty to thirty minutes talking. This will be the single best gift you can give your family, and it will go a long way not only in teaching healthy food habits but bringing you all closer together.

Although it's important to keep your cool when your children don't, it can be impossible in a rushed environment. At the beginning of your transition to longer meals, set a timer for twenty minutes, then thirty. This will teach your rushers to slow down and your picky eater to start eating. If your picky eater does not finish his meal in the half hour allotted, and he is not eating when the timer goes off, excuse him from the table with the explanation that when he is hungry again, you will serve him his dinner. No snacks will be eaten until dinner is finished.

Tip #2: Distinguish between truth and manipulation at the table.

One of most challenging aspects of parenting is to know when to push and when to back off at the table. Do you trust that your child has had enough to eat when she pushes away from the table and says, "I am full"? This essential question is the source of much stress for all parents of picky eaters. It is also the area that many researchers and nutritionists fight over. Many recommend always believing your child, but I advise you to check it out first.

"I am full" can mean many things, such as:

- "I want ice cream and cookies, not my broccoli." (The *Junk-Food Junkie*)

- "Just because I liked chicken last week doesn't mean I like it tonight." (*Dr. Jekyll & Mr. Hyde*)

- "I don't like that my peas have touched my mashed potatoes." (The *Toucher*)

- "I actually am full because I would rather eat many smaller meals and snacks throughout the day than sit and eat a big meal." (The *Grazer*)

- "I want pizza and not the chicken you served." (The *Short Order Diner*)

- "I have never eaten anything that looks like this." (The *Neophyte*)

- "I just want to drink my chocolate milk until I'm full." (The *Drinker*)

> When children eat processed food, they can no longer count on their body to say "stop" because the excess sugar and salt in these products trick the brain into wanting more and more.

- "I am full because I just ate a ton of snacks before dinner." (The *Snacker*)

- "I only want spaghetti with butter or chicken nuggets and nothing else." (*Mr./Miss Bland*)

- "I have a hard time sitting still and just want to get up from the table and play." (The *Player*)

- "I think I may have spotted something gross under my chicken." (The *Inspector*)

- "I can't eat my meal without ketchup on everything." (The *Dipper*)

So as you can see, "I am full" is not as simple as it may seem. Also, when children eat processed food, they can no longer count on their body to say "stop" because the excess sugar and salt in these products trick the brain into wanting more and more. In today's world, you are being asked to believe that children have the ability to know when they are full. They would if served a diet full of whole foods. The reality, though, is that children's diets are made up of too much junk food and thus, "I am full" cannot be trusted at face value any longer.

Many parents are fearful of overfeeding their children. They do not want to override their children's innate ability to regulate their intake of food, and they are afraid they will be contributing to their children developing an eating disorder. When parents with these beliefs hear their children say "I am full," they quickly back away.

These concerns are there for a good reason. Certain messages stick in our heads because we have heard them so many times from professionals and friends: "Do not push or encourage your child to eat." "Back away at the table or you will cause an eating disorder." "Let your children decide how much they are going to eat."

There is no need to be anxious about asking your children whether they are truly full because there is a lot of space between encouraging and forcing when working with children at the table. You can rest assured in knowing that there are plenty of opportunities to encourage your picky eater to take, for instance, two more bites, once you realize that only a truly hungry child will eat and that to get a child who is truly full to continue eating takes a big effort. Questioning their fullness or encouraging children to continue to eat is a far cry from force-feeding them.

THE APPETITE CYCLE

Children's appetites wax and wane throughout their childhood. This natural increase and decrease in appetite makes it difficult to determine whether children are just trying to get out of eating the healthy stuff or whether they just truly do not feel like eating because they are not hungry.

Here are some issues that would cause an increase in appetite:

- Going through a growth spurt
- Exercising a lot during the day
- Missing snacks
- Eating little at the previous meal
- Experiencing anxiety or emotional upset
- Making up for eating little the day before

These issues may cause decrease in appetite:

- Snacking a lot before their meal
- Not feeling well physically or emotionally
- A slow-down in growth
- One of many other valid internal reasons that causes children's appetites to wax and wane from day to day

This may sound like a lot of information to process when deciding whether to encourage your picky eater to keep eating. In reality, this decision is just another example in an endless list of decisions that you make every day while taking into consideration at least a dozen factors, boundaries, and expectations.

The options you have at hand when your child says "I am full" are:

- Believe him immediately and excuse him from the table.
- Check in and ask whether she is sure that she is full, or does she think she could take another couple of bites.
- Excuse him from the table but let him know that when he is hungry again, this food will be making a reappearance.

The best ways I know how to test whether children are full are any of the following statements:

- "You are full? Okay, it's too bad you will not have room for dessert." This usually gets them screaming, "No, I have room!"
- "Okay, I understand that you are full. You can be excused, just know that the next time you are hungry, what you didn't eat for mealtime will be served again." Some children will be fine with this and some will not. Children who are really full should not be forced to finish, and those who are still hungry may eat some more later on.
- "Okay, I'll just wrap this up for later. You can eat it at snack time or for lunch at school tomorrow." That way you are not pressuring your child to eat, but he gets the message loud and clear that he will not be getting snacks and treats in place of a meal.

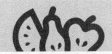

You know your children best, so follow up with a statement that contains these two elements:

1 A confirmation that you heard what they said: "I hear you say that you are full," followed by . . .

2 A consequence that leads to the fact that this food will be eaten if they are not full. (You will know this because they will be asking for a snack within an hour of their meal.) "You can be excused but know that you will not be getting anything else to eat until the next meal." Or, if they did not eat enough healthy food that day: "Okay, but next time you are hungry you need to finish your meal because you did not have enough vegetables and protein today." You are basically calling their bluff or confirming that they are full.

At the end of this chapter, you will learn how much of each food group they should be eating every day. Armed with this information, you can begin to set realistic expectations at mealtime.

Knowing this, you will be better prepared the next time you hear your child say he is full. You will take a breath and check out the validity of that statement before reacting and believing it at face value. Force is never permitted at the table, but encouragement and questioning are always appropriate.

Below are questions to ask yourself when making the decision to take your child at his word when he says that he is full:

1 Has he eaten enough to satisfy his daily requirements?

2 Did he eat a lot of food the day before?

3 Has he come to the table full from snacks?

4 Is he not feeling well, emotionally or physically?

5 Was the portion size appropriate?

6 Is there something going on that may be calling my picky eater from the table (e.g., a favorite show is on, the dog wants to play, or a favorite toy is in sight)?

7 Does he actually want something else? For example, does your picky eater ask for dessert or a snack within minutes of being excused from the table?

Many families throw away leftovers as if they were garbage, and thus children do not learn that food is actually one of the most precious resources on the planet.

Tip #3: Mirror healthy eating.

Mirror, mirror on the wall, how am I doing with my eating habits?

You may not think that what and how you eat even registers with your children, but it does. You took a questionnaire in the previous chapter to review your own eating habits, so you have an overall impression of how you are doing.

If your diet is not a healthy one at the moment, this news may add a layer of stress to your already busy life—but it doesn't have to. You and your entire family can focus on making one simple change a month to turn everyone's unhealthy eating habits around slowly and without drama. I have created just this type of program for you and your busy family at www.buildhealthykids.com. Learn which eating habits or activity to tackle each month and join others who are turning the health of their families around, one step at a time.

In addition to the quality of your and your spouse's diets, consider the following issues when you think of mirroring:

- **What you eat:** If you eat vegetables, fruit, whole grains, healthy proteins and oils, plus dairy, your diet is looking pretty good as long as you limit the amount of junk food and sweetened beverages that you consume. It is also important to cook at home and limit trips to fast-food establishments. If you give in to the lure of a quick drive-through for doughnuts or French fries, your children will grow up to do the same thing.

- **How much you eat:** When you sit down to a meal or snack, do you stop when you are full or do you push past fullness and overeat? Do you finish a bag of cookies or go for several bowls of ice cream after dinner? Do your children hear you say "I am full" and push away from the table? Do you often sit and mindlessly munch a whole bag of chips while watching TV? All of these situations teach your child how they should eat, whether they should listen to their own body or push past satiety and eat too much.

- **How you eat:** When you sit down to eat, are you mindful and focused on eating or rushed and gobble and go? Your children will take your cue on this. If you value mealtime, your children will learn to take a break to eat, too. But if you pay little to no thought of eating and see it as something you have to get over with, your children will behave the same way,

- **Why you eat:** Do you just eat when you are hungry or do you reach for candy or ice cream when you are feeling stressed, sad, or angry? If you turn to food to comfort yourself, your children will learn that they can use food to settle their emotions, too. If you currently use food as your drug of choice, it is not too late to turn this habit around and learn a new way as your children do. The next time you are visibly stressed, angry, or sad, grab your kids and go for a walk, play a game of tag, or catch a baseball.

- **Whether you value food:** Is food something that you respect and think of as a precious resource, or is it something that you easily discard? Many families throw away leftovers as if they were garbage, and thus children do not learn that food is actually one of the most precious resources on the planet and without it we would not survive.

Here are some ways to bring back the value of food to your family:

- Take your children shopping and point out the cost of food. Teach them that even though a bag of chips may be inexpensive, the cost of food goes beyond just the price tag (e.g., look for how many nutrients that dollar can purchase). You can always buy food with little to no nutrition for dirt-cheap. It costs more money to buy foods packed with life-giving nutrition, but by focusing on cutting coupons, stocking up on sale items, and buying in season and bulk items, it doesn't have to be a lot more.

- The next time you have leftovers, bring your children into the kitchen to help you store them in containers and talk about what you are going to do with them tomorrow night for dinner. Teach your children how to transform leftovers, which highlights the value of food. Talk to them repeatedly about how one does not throw away food unless it is expired or rotten, and that as a family, you all will take the time to serve it again.

- Cook with your children. Talk about where the food comes from, which foods were passed down through your family's heritage, and the importance of cherished family recipes. This will help to make food personal for your children. Nothing says "I value food" to children more than letting them see you take time out of your busy day to cook a wholesome meal instead of putting a bag of fast food in front of them.

  Do not worry if you have no idea how to cook. There are dozens of websites and blogs out there that focus on healthy cooking for the family, complete with meal ideas for the week and grocery lists to accompany it. Turn on the Food Network or the Cooking Channel and watch some cooking shows together. Many kids love to watch these types of shows.

- Think about where the food comes from when you sit down to dinner. It is a fun and eye-opening exercise to talk about how that potato got on your child's plate and who to be thankful for: The farmer who planted and picked it, the people who packed it, those who delivered it to your local grocery store, the clerk who put it in the produce aisle, the checkout clerk who rang you up, the parents who worked hard to buy it, and finally whoever prepared the mashed potatoes that now sit in front of you. With awareness and a moment of appreciation, your children will learn this valuable lesson: Food is a precious resource that needs to be treated with respect. Use this example and play "How did it get here?" with your children as often as you want.

- Watch great movies about food and how precious it is, where it comes from, and why it is so essential that we protect our farms and farmers. *Food Inc.* is one example but it is rated PG, so review it first before showing it to your younger child.

- Go to a farmers market or local farm and meet some of the hard workers who bring food to your table and see how much work it takes to actually grow food.

Tip #4: Know what your child's daily food requirements are.

The components of a healthy meal are pictured on the plate below. Half your children's meals should consist of vegetables and fruit, with there being more vegetables than fruit. One quarter of the plate should be a grain (preferably whole grain), and the remaining quarter of the plate should have a source of protein.

A glass of milk completes the meal. How much of each component depends on your child, discussed in the following information about portions.

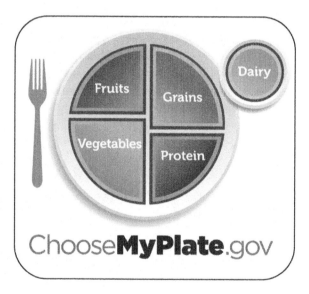

Source: www.choosemyplate.gov

If your children are not eating any one of the five essential food group elements or they have not had enough of a certain food group before mealtime, then let them know that they need to finish it now or it will be served the next time that they are hungry. Better yet, serve the missing component first and when they finish that, serve the rest of the meal. Here is a common scene: Your children sit down to eat dinner, and you know that they have eaten no vegetables until now. They eat their dinner but refuse their broccoli. What do you do?

1 Ask them to eat their broccoli.

2 If that doesn't work, use the "Eat then treat" rule: If you do not eat your broccoli you cannot have dessert.

3 If that doesn't work, excuse them from the table with the understanding that the broccoli will be making a reappearance if they are hungry again before bedtime: "You've had no vegetables today and because vegetables provide the superpowers you need to grow up big and strong (or, depending your child's age, they are essential for meeting your potential), you may not have a snack or dessert until your broccoli is eaten." For dinner the next night, serve the broccoli first before the rest of the meal.

What Serving Size Is Right for My Child?

With the awareness that fluctuations in appetite are normal and keeping in mind the information described previously to distinguish true hunger, it is time to discover what the recommended serving sizes are for children. The U.S. Department of Agriculture (USDA) sets guidelines as to how much food your child should eat in a day. The amounts of food and beverages are based on your children's height, weight, age, and activity level. A table that generalizes the amount of food in each food group that your child needs based on just his or her age and gender and with the assumption that they are getting thirty minutes of moderate exercise a day is included in Appendix B on page 177.

To find out more specific guidelines, go to www.choosemyplate.gov/myplate/index.aspx, where you will discover how much and which types of food your children need based on their actual height, weight, gender, age, and activity level, instead of an average.

Serving Sizes Versus Portions

Don't be fooled by the serving sizes you see on bottles, boxes, jars, and cans. The Nutrition Facts label on the back of most processed foods is based on a 2,000-calorie diet. Many younger children eat much less than this, and many teenage boys will eat more than 2,000 calories in a day.

The serving sizes on the Nutrition Facts label are not recommendations for how much your children should eat. Rather, they are based on portions commonly eaten in each food category. Because children's daily caloric intake varies widely, use the Nutrition Facts label as a general guide only and increase or decrease the amounts based on your child's total caloric needs. Refer to the portion sizes below to learn how much your child should eat at one time.

The Nutrition Facts label is useful when comparing one food to the another—for example, one brand of cereal's sugar content to another. It is also great when looking to see whether a food or beverage is high or low in certain nutrients; the Daily Value (%DV) lets you know how much of the daily intake of a specific nutrient that food is providing, with 5% DV or less being low and 20% DV or more considered high.

What Does a Serving Look Like?

Here are some common sizes:

- ¼ cup is the size of a large egg.

- ½ cup is the size of half of either a baseball or tennis ball.

- 1 cup is the size of an adult fist or baseball.

Specifics on Servings Sizes for Each Food Group

The USDA has determined how much food and beverages your children need to consume to be healthy. The food is broken into groups of fruits, vegetables, dairy, grains, oils, and proteins like meat or beans. There is also a category called "empty calories," which takes into account the leftover calories for added solid fats and sugar in children's diets after children have consumed their required fruits, vegetables, protein, dairy, grains, and fat.

The following sections explain how much of each of these food groups your picky eater needs on a daily basis. If your child follows a restricted diet because of allergies, sensitivities, other medical conditions, or belief systems, work with a nutritionist to determine what your child's daily intake should be.

Grains

Children need two to seven servings of grain a day measured in ounce equivalents depending on their total caloric requirement (see Appendix B). Although the USDA suggests that at least half the grain servings be whole grains, I suggest going even further and making all your children's grains whole grains.

Depending on your children's appetite, the following is the typical serving size of grains at a sitting (the USDA uses a unit of measure for grains called ounce equivalent):

- Children age two: ½ ounce equivalent = ½ cup (14 g) of cold cereal, ½ slice of bread, or ¼ muffin

- Children ages three to six: 1 ounce equivalent = 1 mini bagel, 1 slice bread, ½ muffin, 1 cup (28 g) cold cereal, or ½ cup (40 g) hot cereal, (70 g) pasta, or (98 g) rice

- Children ages seven to approximately nine: 1½ ounces equivalent = 1½ slices of bread, 1½ cups (42 g) cold cereal, or ¾ cup (60 g) hot cereal, (105 g) pasta, or (146 g) rice

- Children ages ten and older: 2 ounces equivalent = ½ large bagel, 1 muffin, 2 slices regular size bread, 2 cups (56 g) cold cereal, or 1 cup (80 g) hot cereal, (140 g) pasta, or (195 g) rice

If children are hungry after one serving, by all means give them another as long as they have eaten the fruit, vegetable, and protein servings that are also on their plate. Try to stick to the daily servings of grains because many children will ask for more and more carbohydrates (grains) at meals or snack time and leave the vegetables or fruit to the side and maybe the protein, too. This is where the "eat then treat" rule works very well. It look like this: "Finish your vegetables and then I'll give you more pasta." The pasta becomes the lure.

Fruit

Children's daily requirement for fruit, which also includes juice, is 1 to 2 cups a day (see Appendix B for specific amounts). It is better for your children to eat their fruit than to drink it because the whole fruit provides all the nutrients plus the fiber that is lacking in juice. If you do serve juice to your children, limit it to ½ cup (120 ml) for two- to six-year-olds and 1 cup (235 ml) for children seven years and older.

Following are typical serving sizes of fruit at a sitting:

- Children age two: ¼ cup = 2 inches (5 cm) of a banana (cut up, of course), or ¼ cup (60 g) applesauce

- Children ages three to six years: ½ cup = 4 inches (10 cm) of a banana, ½ cup (125 g) applesauce, 16 grapes, ½ small apple, 1 small peach, 1 plum, 1 small orange, or ¼ cup (35 g) raisins

- Children ages seven to approximately nine years: ¾ cup (184 g) diced fruit, or 6 inches (15 cm) of a banana

- Children ages ten and older: 1 cup = 8 to 9 inches (20 to 22.5 cm) of banana, 2 medium plums, 1 cup (245 g) diced fruit, 1 peach, 1 large orange, 32 grapes, or ½ cup (75 g) raisins

These are average serving sizes, but they give you a figure to work with at meal and snack time. Make sure your children eat a variety of fruit, as many children just stick to apples and bananas. If you buy fruit in cans or frozen, stick to those that say "water added" or "fruit juice-sweetened."

The following do NOT count as a serving of fruit:

• Gummy fruit snacks

• Fruit roll-ups

• Fruit strips

In addition to all of the ill effects that too much sugar brings (discussed in chapter 2), the stickiness of these gummy products keeps dentists very busy. Teach your picky eater the difference between real fruit and candy in disguise.

Vegetables

Children need 1 to 2½ cups of vegetables a day based on their total caloric intake (see Appendix B). Vegetables are a very important food that children need to eat to reach their potential and prevent diseases later in life. Do not rely on vegetable juice, hiding your children's vegetables in other foods, or giving them gummy vegetable supplements instead of the real thing. Vegetable juice and supplements do not deliver phytonutrients—nutrients specific to plants—in the concentration that they are found in nature. Whenever you concentrate one part of the plant, or the entire plant, you are changing its identity and thus ultimately altering its nutritional profile. It is best to stick to straight-from-nature vegetables.

Following are typical serving sizes of vegetables at a sitting—note that in general, 1 cup of raw or cooked vegetables, or 2 cups of raw leafy greens can be considered as 1 cup from the vegetable group:

• Children age two: ¼ cup = ¼ cup (33 g) carrots, (41 g) corn, or (18 g) broccoli

• Children ages three to six: ½ cup = ½ cup (36 g) broccoli, (65 g) carrots, (82 g) corn; 1 cup (57 g) lettuce leaves, (36 g) kale, or other leafy green; ½ medium potato; 1 small green pepper or tomato

• Children ages seven to approximately nine: ¾ cup = ¾ cup (75 g) cauliflower, (113 g) peas, or (53 g) mushrooms

• Children ages ten and older: 1 cup = 2 cups leafy greens like (134 g) kale, (72 g) collard greens, or (114 g) lettuce; 1 cup (71 g) broccoli, (164 g) corn, (130 g) carrots; 1 medium potato, 1 large green pepper or tomato

Dairy

The dairy requirements for children are 2 to 3 cups a day (see Appendix B). Beyond the age of two, children should only consume dairy products that are low- or non-fat. Between the ages of one and two, the dairy products you serve need to be whole-fat varieties in order to provide these children with the essential fat they need to grow and develop. Stick to unflavored milk because chocolate, vanilla, and strawberry milk add unnecessary sugar to your children's diet.

Following are the typical serving sizes of dairy at a sitting; the USDA defines what 1 cup of dairy equals, which is different than the standard measuring system used in kitchens when referring to cheese products. In general, 1 cup of the dairy requirement counts as 1 cup (235 ml) of milk or (230 g) yogurt and 2 ounces (55 g) of cheese.

- Children age two: ¼ cup = 2 ounces (55 g) yogurt, or ½ cup (115 g) cottage cheese (1 slice of American cheese equals 1/3 cup)

- Children ages three to six: ½ cup = 4 ounces (115 g) yogurt or one slice hard cheese such as cheddar

- Children ages seven to approximately nine: ¾ cup = 6 ounces (170 g) yogurt

- Children ages ten and older: 1 cup = 2 cups (450 g) cottage cheese, 8 ounces (225 g) yogurt, 2 slices hard cheese, 3 slices American cheese

For children who are dairy intolerant, make sure they are drinking and eating foods and beverages high in calcium each day in amounts equal to the missing dairy requirements. Also, work with a nutritionist to make sure your children are getting enough protein, calcium, potassium, and vitamin D, which are also found in dairy products.

Protein Sources

Most children in the United States get enough protein from their diet. Children and adults can improve the quality of their protein intake, however, by getting more vegetable sources of protein such as legumes, limiting red meat, adding fish twice a week, and choosing healthier animal sources such as white meat from poultry.

Children need two to six ½-ounce equivalents in their diet daily (see Appendix B). Following are the typical serving sizes of protein at a sitting:

- Children age two: ½ ounce equivalent, or ½ egg, ½ ounce (15 g) of meat

- Children ages three to six: 1 ounce equivalent, or 1 tablespoon (16 g) peanut butter, 12 almonds, ½ cup (120 ml) lentil soup, 2 tablespoons (31 g) hummus, 1 egg, 1 sandwich slice of turkey, or 1 ounce (28 g) cooked chicken, lean beef, or lean pork

- Children ages seven to approximately nine: 2 ounces equivalent, or 1 cup (235 ml) lentil or split pea soup, ½ cup (89 g) kidney beans, 1 soy or bean patty, 1 ounce (28 g) nuts or seeds, or 2 eggs

- Children ages ten and older: 2 to 3 ounces equivalent, or 1 small chicken breast, 1 can tuna, or 1 small cooked lean hamburger

In general, 1 ounce of meat, poultry, or fish; ¼ cup (25 g) cooked dry beans; 1 egg; 1 tablespoon (16 g) of peanut butter; or ½ ounce of nuts or seeds equals one 1-ounce equivalent for protein.

Focus on making sure that your children get two servings of fish, three to four servings of legumes at a minimum, and no more than one serving of red meat each week. You can fill in the rest of the meals with poultry, low-fat cheese dishes, and vegetarian options.

Focus on making sure that your children get two servings of fish, three to four servings of legumes at a minimum, and no more than one serving of red meat each week.

Oils

Your children need 3 to 6 teaspoons of oil a day. Many children get enough unhealthy solid fat from baked products, whole-milk dairy products, beef, and butter. Your focus is on making sure that your children's diet provides a healthy source of essential fatty acids while being low in solid/saturated fats—more vegetable oils and less butter and whole-milk products, for example. Here's a handy visual:

- 1 teaspoon of margarine or butter = a finger tip

- 2 tablespoons (28 g) salad dressing = size of a Ping-Pong ball

You are now ready to dig deep into your child's unique eating personalities. Under the term *picky eater*, there are many, many faces. In section 2, you will learn how the temperament that your child is born with affects his or her relationship with food and also discover specific picky eating personalities. You are sure to recognize your picky eater in some of the descriptions that follow.

CHAPTER 5

Nine Temperaments at the Table—Learn What Makes Your Child Tick

Each child is born with different behavioral traits for dealing with the world. These innate traits are called temperaments, which refer to a child's style of interacting with people, places, and things—and, for the purpose of this book, food. A group of physicians and researchers started to investigate the concept of temperaments in children in the mid-1950s and identified nine different temperament traits that babies are born with that remain relatively stable throughout a child's life. Today the concept of the nine temperaments is widely accepted.

Once you are able to understand your child's temperament traits, you will have a much easier time parenting your child, especially at the table. You cannot change your child's temperament, but you can learn how to handle your child effectively at the table and beyond.

Each of the nine temperaments is present in every child to varying degrees. Some children will be born with high degrees of one trait, others a low level of the same trait, while most others fall somewhere in between. Your child's temperament has a large influence when it comes to how he or she approaches food.

Before you start blaming yourself, what you ate during pregnancy, or the time you yelled out of frustration, know with certainty that you did not make your child shy about trying new foods or stubborn in his or her ways. Biologically based temperaments drive this behavior. The good news is that although temperaments remain relatively stable over time, they can be influenced a little based on a child's experiences, environment, interactions with other people, and health.

These temperaments are the basis of the five eating personalities that you will learn about in the next chapter. The chart below lists the nine temperaments and how they are manifested at the table.

Temperament trait	How it manifests at the table
• Sensitivity	• Highly sensitive to food and the environment; rejects many "new" foods at first.
• Distractibility	• Highly focused: hard to get to the table when absorbed in an activity. • Easily distracted: doesn't pay attention to the meal, leaves the table often.
• Activity level	• Active: leaves the table often; can't sit still.
• Intensity	• Low reactors need encouragement to eat. • Strong reactors pitch a fit when served a food they don't want.
• Adaptability	• Slow to accept a new food; may take more than 12 exposures to "like" a new food.
• Approach or withdrawal	• Slow to approach a new food.
• Persistence	• Very persistent eaters will keep asking for a food until you give in. • Easily frustrated eaters stop eating quickly if the slightest thing is out of the norm.
• Regularity	• Eaters with regular schedules. • Eaters without routine schedules.
• Quality of mood	• Negative eaters easily find problems with their meal and the environment.

Answer the questions in the quizzes below to determine where your child lands on the scale (high, low, or in the middle) for each of the nine temperaments so that you can better understand what makes him or her tick at the table. There are no right or wrong answers, so be honest in your assessment.

Step 1: Determine where your child falls on the picky eating scale.

Take the following quiz to determine whether your child is a picky eater or suffers from the disorder known as sensory food aversion, discussed previously.

A picky eater can be managed at home with the tools, information, and advice presented in this book. Children with sensory disorders, however, need some backup from an occupational or speech therapist because the sensory system in their body does not support their eating or drinking process adequately. These children will resist eating to the point where their health is at risk. Do not miss this essential information. Answer yes or no to the following questions.

The Picky Eating Scale

1 **Has your child been diagnosed with a developmental delay, Asperger's, autism, ADHD, or other behavioral or psychiatric condition?**

2 **Does your child insist that one or more than one food be present at every meal?**

3 **Does your child overreact (e.g., finds most smells overwhelming) or underreact (e.g., he can't smell a thing because he is always congested with colds or allergies) to smells?**

4 **Does your child get visibly anxious (e.g., shake, cry, throw a tantrum) when presented with a new food?**

5 **Does your child eat fifteen or fewer foods on a regular basis?**

6 **Does your child gag or vomit often when eating a new food or a food she does not want to eat?**

7 **Does your child refuse to consume *any* of the following food groups: fruit, vegetable, protein, grains, or dairy/dairy alternative?**

8 **Does your child resist food to such a degree that he never gives in and tries a bite or finishes his meal? For example, he will go to bed without eating his dinner if asked to eat a food he does not want to eat?**

9 **Does this sentence describe your child? My child does not get used to new foods after a dozen attempts and remains resistant over time no matter how many times I present the food.**

10 **Does your child drop or spill food and drinks often?**

The degree to which your child is picky about eating food can range from normal to resistant. Count the number of times you answered yes to the questions above to determine where on the scale below your child falls.

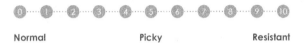

Normal   Picky   Resistant

If you answered no to all the questions above, then your child scored normal on the picky eating scale.

If you answered yes to many (more than five) of the questions or if you answered yes to questions 1, 4, and 6, you need to follow up with your child's pediatrician.

If you answered yes to some (five or fewer) of the questions, your child is most likely a picky eater, and you can follow the advice in this book without backup. However, if you have any hesitation or concern, check with your child's pediatrician to rule out a sensory disorder.

Step 2: Discover your child's temperament.

Now let's start the fun. Learn how your child's temperament influences his or her behavior toward food by taking a quiz on each of the nine following temperament traits and discover how best to work with each. If your child scores high on any difficult aspect of these temperaments, you may only need to work with his or her innate tendencies to turn your picky eater around.

1. Sensitivity

Sensitivity refers to how easily a child is disturbed by changes in his or her environment. It can also be viewed as the amount of stimulation you need to give your child to elicit a response. A very sensitive child needs little provocation to react to food, environment, texture, or taste, whereas a child with little to no sensitivity around food does not react to different tastes, textures, and environments and will be much easier to feed.

1 **How sensitive is your child to the temperature of his food or drink?**

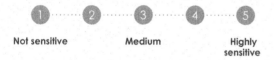

2 **How sensitive is your child to the texture of her food (e.g., she will not eat anything but pureed food, doesn't like the feeling of the chunks of food in soups and pasta)?**

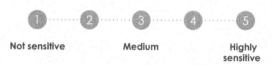

3 **How sensitive is your child to new foods and drinks?**

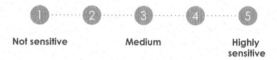

4 **Is your child able to distinguish different subtle flavors in foods or know immediately if you changed brands?**

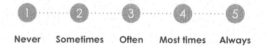

5 **How sensitive is your child to lights or sounds in his environment?**

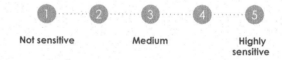

Highly sensitive children are difficult to feed, as they usually have only a select number of foods that they will eat and they will often resist any new food.

If answering any of the questions was difficult or if you never really thought about the issues in question, read the following section to be able to identify whether your child has a sensitivity issue. Many picky eaters do have a sensitivity issue, but parents lump their children into the "picky eater" category and look no further. This is understandable, as feeding a picky eater can be so overwhelming at times it is difficult for anyone in the day-to-day struggle to pick apart what aspects of eating may be giving their child a hard time.

If your children scored a total of 16 or above, they would be considered a sensitive eater; so would scoring a 4 or more on any of the questions. Your child may be sensitive to one aspect of a food or drink—the texture and not the taste, for example, or just the temperature. In these cases, you will still need to use the strategies laid out below to turn around your sensitive eater. Read the following section to both discover whether your child is a sensitive eater and if so, how to work with him or her.

Strategies to Help the Highly Sensitive Eater

Highly sensitive children are difficult to feed, as they usually have only a select number of foods that they will eat and they will often, if not always, resist any new food. If you did not have a clue that your child was sensitive to food, you most likely found feeding him or her to be extremely stressful. The foods and beverages your sensitive child prefers may seem random to you, but once you understand what aspect of a food or drink is giving your child a rough time, you will be better able to handle his or her sensitivity at the table.

Start by slowly beginning to work with, not against, their predispositions. Change one aspect of a food at a time. For example, if your child has an issue with colors and shapes of a food, serve her foods that she is comfortable with and add one new color to her plate at a time.

If your child has multiple food sensitivity issues or you cannot put your finger on which aspects are bothersome, keep everything the same while you change one aspect of the food. For example, you wouldn't add a hard, crunchy orange carrot to the diet of a child who currently eats mostly white foods that are soft and bland. You may consider adding a different colored bland food like mashed orange sweet potatoes, for example.

Encourage your sensitive eater to broaden his palate and the amount of foods he will eat by introducing one new food at a time. Present the new food multiple times, encourage him to eat it, have him see you eating it, and use the reward system if necessary. You may also consider serving the new food in your son's favorite bowl or plate. If he does not have one, go out and buy one for him so that he can find comfort and familiarity in what his food is served on.

If you do not have a sensitive temperament, then you may find yourself thinking that your child is overreacting and in return become angry because you think she is "overdoing it." This reaction only serves to push an already volatile situation with a highly sensitive child closer to the edge. Your job as a parent to a sensitive child is to teach her to express her reactions and feelings in a more socially appropriate way. Take a deep breath: Remind yourself that your child is hardwired to overreact; listen and acknowledge her strong feelings; and end with several more appropriate options that she could have used.

If your child is very sensitive to food, he is most likely sensitive to other things in his environment such as the sounds, sights, and smells around him. In addition to discovering the aspects of food that aggravate your sensitive child, observe him eating in different environments to determine whether sound (loud music or the television), energy (chaos versus calm), and sights (bright or flickering lights) set him up to not be able to eat his meal because he is busy trying to assimilate all the environmental attacks to his senses. Create a calm and centering environment for your sensitive eater, as discussed in chapter 4. This calm environment will also help you to be able to keep it together when eating with your sensitive eater.

And last, do not let your child hear you call him or her a picky or sensitive eater. These terms convey judgment and disapproval, which adds nothing positive to your child's eating behaviors. It can also be a self-fulfilling prophecy whereby you are so intent on looking for when she is a picky, sensitive eater that you miss out on praising your child when she is not. Use any of the following statements instead: "You certainly know what you like," "You have supersonic taste buds," or "You may grow up to be a chef one day with your ability to taste food so well."

Use his sensitivity to your advantage by asking your child to help you prepare food: "Should I use more garlic in here?" "Do you think this sauce needs more flavor?" or "Which brand of bread do you prefer and why?" Asking your child to articulate why it is he prefers some food or brand to another will give you clues to what drives him when selecting the foods he will and will not eat.

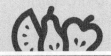

DETERMINING WHETHER YOUR CHILD IS A SENSITIVE EATER

The first step in unraveling the mystery of your picky eater is to notice whether there are similarities in the foods or beverages that your child does not like by writing down which ones he will not consume over a four-day period. Follow up by noticing whether there are common aspects to these foods and beverages: For example, are they creamy, chunky, thick, watery, hot, cold, crunchy, mushy, spicy, or bland? Any one of these characteristics may aggravate or appeal to your sensitive eaters depending upon the "sense" that they have an issue with:

- Taste: prefers bland or spicy food

- Touch: prefers textured or smooth foods; prefers hot or cold foods and beverages

- Sight: wants foods in the same shape or color

- Smell: prefers foods with either a strong or limited smell

- Sound: prefers foods that make no sound or that make a lot of sound, like crunchy foods

Below are other issues highly sensitive eaters face and ways to work with these challenges. If this seems too complicated to you, contact an occupational or speech therapist to help.

Issue	Solution
They avoid mixing textures or foods like mashed potatoes and gravy.	Serve each food separately.
They do not like it when one food touches another.	Purchase a plate that has sections so their foods are kept separate. (Read about the *Toucher*.)
They need each meal and snack to be predictable and without surprises.	Purchase or use their favorite plate, cup, and bowl at each meal, plus tell them beforehand what you are serving.
They eat so much of a food that they will no longer eat it anymore.	Make sure your child does not eat the same food at each meal or the same meal three days in a row.

2. Distractibility

Distractibility refers to how easily a child is sidetracked from the current activity (eating) by outside stimuli. On one end of the distractibility spectrum is "easily distracted," and at the other is "extreme focus." A child who is extremely focused on one task, for example, may need extra encouragement to come to the table.

1 **When eating a meal or snack, how easily is your child distracted by noises, people, toys, or events?**

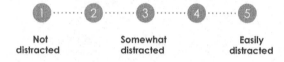

Not distracted   Somewhat distracted   Easily distracted

2 **Does your child stop eating when, for example, a sibling leaves the table, the family pet enters the room, or the phone starts to ring?**

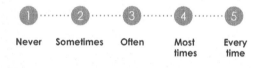

Never   Sometimes   Often   Most times   Every time

3 **Does your child find it difficult to focus on eating when others are at the table? Does he talk excessively, for example, to the point whereby he does not eat his meal?**

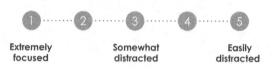

Extremely focused   Somewhat distracted   Easily distracted

4 **Is your child easily distracted with items on the table during meal and snack time? Does she play with her utensils and other items on the table instead of eating the meal, for example?**

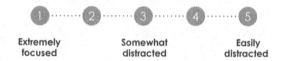

Extremely focused   Somewhat distracted   Easily distracted

This distractibility trait makes it difficult for a child to register internal cues that may be saying "I am hungry" or "I am full."

Strategies to Help the Highly Focused Eater

If your children scored a 6 or below, he is very focused on the task at hand and hard to distract. The highly focused child at the table will not have as many difficulties when it comes to eating as a highly distractible child, but there are still several issues to consider with this type of child. Transition time may be especially challenging for highly focused children if they are also highly focused when playing: You may have a difficult time getting them to the table because they do not want to stop playing to come to dinner.

Getting a highly focused child to the table will take preparation and warning. The best thing that you can do is to set a timer to ring five minutes before dinnertime. This will alert your child that he needs to wrap things up and get ready to eat. A highly focused child may also need a gentle touch and eye contact to break his attention away from what he is currently doing. Talk to your child as you approach so that you do not startle him. Place your hand on his shoulder while you announce "It is dinnertime." Gently turn the child to face you while you let him know what is expected of him and say, "We are going to be eating in five minutes. Please clean up your toys and come to the table after you wash your hands."

If you are a quick mover and thinker, you may find yourself easily frustrated with your focused child. Take some deep breaths to calm and center yourself while remembering that your focused child was born that way and will excel in areas that require concentration. Use those brief moments to attend to yourself. Everyone will be better off if you do.

Strategies to Help the Easily Distracted Eater

If your child scored 13 or above, then you have an issue with distractability at the table. This inability to focus on the task at hand (eating) can easily turn into a child who leaves the table before she has had enough to eat, or the child may eat too much because she is not paying attention to the meal. This distractibility trait makes it difficult for a child to register internal cues that may be saying "I am hungry" or "I am full." Because of this, paying attention to appropriate serving sizes is necessary to make sure an easily distracted child is getting enough, and not too much, to eat.

Easily distracted children may not notice subtle changes in the taste and texture of food. This may serve you well if your child is a picky eater, as you can easily distract him with a story or movement so that you can get food into him. For example, when feeding an easily distracted toddler, you may have difficulty getting him to focus on eating his meal but you can just as easily say, "Look at this" while you give him a bite of a new vegetable.

The most important technique for these children is to limit distractions around them while they are eating. Try these methods:

- Have your child eat at the dining room or kitchen table; eating in the living room or playroom is asking for trouble, as your child will want to play or watch television instead of eat.

- Follow the advice in chapter 4 about setting the stage. Remove toys from the table unless you are using them as a bribe, plus keep salt and pepper shakers as well as other items out of your child's reach.

- If your child does become distracted, teach him or her how to deal with it at the table: "I noticed you heard the dog bark. Fluffy is fine. Go back to eating please," or "That salt shaker looks like a toy but instead of playing with it, tell me a story starring Super Salty," and then have everyone add on a scene or two.

- Because the easily distracted child has difficulty sitting still for extended periods, break up mealtime into smaller, easier-to-manage, episodes. Here's how:

  - Set a timer for two to five minutes, depending on your child's ability to focus, and have your child come to the table and sit for that length of time.

  - After the initial time period let your child have a break for two to three minutes; call her back again for another brief eating episode and continue this until she has finished her meal or is truly full.

  - Praise your child each time he is able to sit and focus at the table. Slowly increase the table time until you have trained your easily distracted child to eat his entire meal without a break.

You can also consider using your children's distractibility as a tool for a brief period until you have trained them to sit and eat a meal: Tell them they can play with their toy at the table as long as they take one more bite. Remove the toy if they stop eating and continue this until they have eaten an appropriate portion. Use whichever method works best for your children—table breaks or allowing toys at the table. The solution will also depend on whether your sensitive child has siblings. You need to choose a solution that works for your entire family.

Highly distracted children will have a difficult time eating when they go out to a restaurant. It is best if you can limit your trips to eat out to a minimum—realize that your highly distractible children cannot "stop" noticing even the slightest smells, sounds, and movements in their immediate environment.

Consider feeding your easily distracted child before you go out to eat so at least you know that he has consumed the healthy food that he needs. You can also take a break between courses by either going outside or walking your easily distracted child to the bathroom to stretch his legs and look around. As a last resort, you may need to turn on an electronic device to keep your child occupied so at least the rest of the family can eat in peace. Only use an electronic device as a last resort and infrequently or else your child will use his misbehaving as a way to play electronics at the table.

Last, remember that your child has no control over how easily distracted she is. Try to see, smell, and hear the world through her eyes, nose, and ears. It can be very overwhelming at times to be easily distracted, and it was not a choice your child made. Presenting yourself in a calm manner will help to settle your distractible child; throwing more things at her to distract her may work in the short term but does not teach her how to work with his tendency to notice everything around her in the long term.

3. Activity Level

This temperament trait focuses on your child's body movements and refers to his physical energy level. Is your child always on the move, or does he like to sit and read for most of the day? On one end of the spectrum with this trait, you have a child who cannot sit still even for a moment, and at the other end, a couch potato. In regard to mealtime, you want to look at how much your child's body moves when she is eating. This temperament quiz will assess whether your child's physical activity level interferes with his eating a healthy diet.

1 **Does your child fidget or have trouble sitting still at mealtime?**

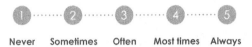

2 **Does your child get up and down from his chair multiple times during a meal?**

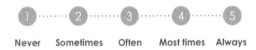

3 **Do you have a hard time getting your child to stay seated long enough to finish eating?**

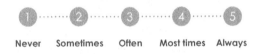

4 **Would your child rather walk or run around with his food than sit down to eat?**

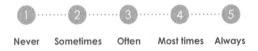

If your child scored 12 to 15 points, he is moderately active and his activity level may interfere with his diet. A score of 16 or higher means that your child's physical energy level is definitely high enough to interfere with his ability to consume sufficient nutrients at mealtime. Follow the strategies listed for your active child.

Strategies to Help the Active Eater

It is best to work with, instead of against, your child's high activity level. Understanding that your child is hardwired to be physically active throughout the day will help you to understand that he is not being difficult, his body is just built to move around a lot.

Your active child may very well do better with eating smaller meals and healthy snacks than having to sit for long periods during meals. As long as your active child is consuming healthy food and beverages for meals and snacks, this will not be a problem. If, however, your active eater eats little at meals and focuses instead on snack foods that tend to be less nutritious, then you do have an issue that you need to work on. Follow the strategies below to extend mealtime enough to ensure that your active eater gets enough nutritious food for his or her growth and health.

- Set realistic goals for your fidgeter to follow. Break down mealtime into "bite episodes." Young children (under 4 years) are often overwhelmed when they sit down to a full meal, but if you ask them to take three bites, you will often be greeted with a smile. Tell your active child that you expect her to eat three bites at the table, and then she can be excused. Allow her to walk around or play quietly with the understanding that she needs to come back in a couple of minutes for three more bites. Set a timer for two minutes with the understanding that when it goes off she needs to come back to the table immediately. Once your child is used to the three-bite goal, you can increase it to four bites and then five bites until she is eating an entire meal without breaks.

- If your child snacks often between meals on healthy food, then you can lower your expectations for how much your child needs to consume at mealtime.

- For a child older than five years, set a timer for five minutes when he gets to the table. Let him know that at the end of five minutes he may leave the table for three minutes but then must return for another five minutes. Once your active older (five years and up) child is comfortable with this, increase his table time by one minute (still keep the breaks to three minutes) until he is able to finish his meal.

- Do not allow any electronics or phone or text time during the breaks. You want to still preserve mealtime, and that means anything that is stimulating is turned off or prohibited.

- Active children need ample opportunities to run, jump, and play throughout the day to get their energy out, especially before mealtimes. Send your children out to play before lunch and dinner. Give them a twenty-minute calm-down period before meals to de-escalate so that they do not come to the table wired.

4. Intensity

This trait refers to the energy level with which your child responds to a situation, whether his reaction is positive or negative. When your child is served his favorite dinner, does he jump up and down with excitement? If so, he is a strong reactor. If, however, he glances at his favorite food and shows little to no response, he would be considered a low reactor.

The intensity that children display at the dinner table is not an issue when a favorite food is served. Quite the contrary, it is when they are served something that they do not want to eat that the problem arises. The strong reactor pitches such a fit that most parents back off. These intense reactors will yell, exclaim "Yuck!", and may even push or throw their food away. No one wants to wrestle with this bear at the table, especially after a long, hard day.

At the other end of the spectrum, low reactors may need a little nudge of encouragement to get them eating. Take the quiz below to determine where your child's intensity score falls.

1 **Does your child scream or react strongly with joy or pleasure when a favorite food is served?**

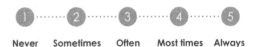

2 **Does your child react strongly when served something that she does not want to eat—for example, yell, scream "Yuck!", leave the table, or push away food?**

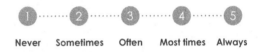

3 **Does your child react strongly, either positively or negatively, when served a new food?**

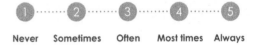

4 **Does your child scare you or make others uncomfortable with his reaction to food at a meal or snack time?**

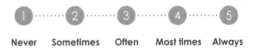

Your child is a low reactor if the score is between 4 and 6 points; is in the middle range of intensity with a score of 7 to 11; and is in the strong reactor category with a score of 12 and above.

If your children yell "Yuck!" or any other negative exclamation at the table, give them one warning and then a time-out if they do not stop.

Strategies to Help the Low Reactor Eater

If your child has little to no reaction when her meal or a new food is placed in front of her, you will need to encourage her to try a few bites to get her initially engaged. You can use a reward system if needed and create a chart with foods and beverages plus amounts that she is expected to eat. She gets a star or points when she eats what is expected.

The low reactor may very likely be the child who "eats to live" and not "lives to eat." You will need to inform your child what is expected from him at the table and why it is important to eat his food: "If you want to grow big and tall like daddy, you need to eat your meal," or "If you want to have the stamina to play soccer well, you need to finish your meal." Because you cannot engage his excitement, work with his cognition—why it is so important to eat his meal. Motivate your child with the facts and set reasonable expectations of how much food he is expected to finish.

Strategies to Help the Strong Reactor Eater

You cannot make strong reactors less reactive but you can help to modify their outbursts and contain them to an appropriate place and time. If your child is a strong reactor, you will need to be prepared for outbursts, especially negative ones. This applies to both an intense reaction to a new food and a negative reaction to a food that the child is accustomed to but does not like very much.

If your child is outspoken and physically demonstrative in a negative fashion, you will want to curtail her response as you would any other inappropriate outburst. Remind your intense reactor that she can let off steam before and after the meal, but she needs to keep it together during mealtime. If she needs a "burst break," excuse her to her room where she can kick and scream before returning to the table.

The environment is crucial for strong reactors. Make sure you have set up meal- and snack time according to the rules outlined in chapter 4. Play soothing music, slightly dim lights, and remove all electronics. Outside stimuli can rev up a strong reactor, so keep things calm and mellow at the table.

If your children yell "Yuck!" or any other negative exclamation at the table, give them one warning and then a time-out if they do not stop. Let them know that "Yuck!" and its variants are not allowed at the table, as discussed chapter 3. If your child reacts by pushing the plate or food away, let him know that this is dinner and you expect him to eat it. If he goes so far as to throw his food, send him immediately to a time-out. When the time-out is over, have him return to the table to eat his meal. If he chooses not to, do not offer another meal and excuse him from the table. When he is hungry, let him know that his dinner will be waiting for him. Note: Use this technique only for children who do not have an emotional or physical issue that prevents them from making informed decisions.

The most effective tool for dealing with strong reactors is to prepare them before the meal or snack. Strong reactors need to react, and it is best if they can let their feelings loose before they sit down at the table, where outbursts are not appropriate behavior. You also do not want them influencing other children; it takes just one "yuck" to ruin everyone's meal.

Before your child gets to the table, let her know what you will be serving so she can get "it" out of her system. When she is screaming or jumping up and down, your job is to listen to her. Try this technique, called Listen, Validate, Inform, Problem-Solve, Sense of Control:

- Let the child know you heard her and validate her feelings: "I understand that you do not want to eat the broccoli. I know it is not your favorite."

- Inform her why the food is so important: "The broccoli is a super food that will help you grow big and strong."

- Problem-solve: "Maybe if you add soy sauce to the broccoli it won't be as bitter."

- Or ask the child for a solution: "What do you think you can do to be able to eat your broccoli?"

- And finally leave her with a sense of control: "Tomorrow night you can pick your favorite vegetable."

This technique works in many situations, so it's worth getting to know and using often with your picky eater.

5. Adaptability

This temperament trait refers to how long it takes for your child to adjust to change over time—not the initial reaction, which is covered later in the "approach/withdrawal" section. If you change your child's brand of peanut butter, does your child still complain weeks later? Does your child have trouble eating at a new babysitter's house or a new preschool? Is transitioning from playing to eating a daily battle in your house? These are issues that slow adapters face. Answer the following questions to determine whether your child is a slow adapter.

1   **Does your child have a hard time or get upset when you ask him to finish up with his current activity to go to the table to eat?**

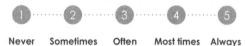

Never   Sometimes   Often   Most times   Always

2   **Does it take your child awhile to adjust to a new eating environment—for example, using a booster seat instead of a high chair, eating lunch at a new school or daycare, or sitting at a different seat at the table?**

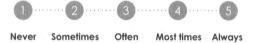

Never   Sometimes   Often   Most times   Always

3   **Does it take your child a long time (more than twelve exposures) to adjust to changes in food—for example, milk instead of juice for lunch, a different brand of peanut butter, or crinkle-cut fries instead of shoestring fries?**

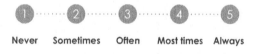

Never   Sometimes   Often   Most times   Always

4   **Have there been a lot of significant changes in your child's environment lately—for example, a new school, new sibling, new home, or new babysitter?**

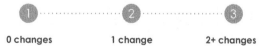

0 changes   1 change   2+ changes

If your child scored a 9 or more on questions 1 through 3, he is a slow adapter. Also, if your child scored 3 or more on question 4, he will be even more sensitive to any slight change in his environment until he gets used to the most recent change.

Strategies to Help the Slow Adapter Eater

Some children take a long time to adjust to a change in their environment, while others accept changes without missing a beat. For those children who are slow to adapt, try to keep changes in their environment to a minimum and add no more than one change at a time if possible. Predictability and routine are essential for the slow adapter, as are more time and support to get used to a new situation, food, or routine.

The best thing you can do when working with slow adapters is to accept and understand how this temperament trait translates into their day-to-day lives. If you try to rush a slow adapter or throw too many changes at her and then get frustrated when she is not moving fast enough, you will be making a manageable situation very stressful for both of you. No matter how frustrated you are with this trait, you will save time and gray hairs by just accepting what is. Your child has no control over needing a longer time than others to adapt to change.

Wait until your child becomes accustomed to one new food before introducing another.

How long it takes for your slow adapter to adjust is up to your individual child, as is finding out what helps her to relax and feel safe again after a change. For example, bring her security blanket or favorite toy to a new school or have her favorite toy sit next to her at mealtime. The only thing you can do to expedite your slow adapter's acceptance of a change is to make the change as comfortable as possible and add no additional changes until the child has grown accustomed to the initial change.

Slow adapters also do better when you take the time to explain to them beforehand what is about to occur. If your slow adapter is eating in a new environment, wait for him to become accustomed to it before introducing a new food or beverage. This is true whether you move schools, change babysitters, or are just trying out a new restaurant. Try to keep everything else the same, such as his usual lunch or beverage. Once your child is settled in, you can begin the process of broadening his diet.

The same holds true for introducing new foods. Wait until your child becomes accustomed to one new food before introducing another. When you want to introduce a new food or beverage, give your slow adapter a heads up so that he can be prepared: "I am going to serve you milk for lunch instead of juice because milk makes you grow big and builds superstrong bones." In this example, make drinking milk a habit at home first before you put it in their lunch box. It is too much to expect them to change their beverage in a chaotic cafeteria setting.

A slow adapter also needs notice long before you expect him to finish one activity and go to another, such as to stop playing and go to the table for lunch. Ten minutes before lunch is served, let your child know that you will be asking him to wrap it up in ten minutes. Follow that with a five-minute warning and then a one-minute warning. Even then, you most likely will need to either guide your child over to the table by gently steering him with your hand or do the time-honored routine of counting: "I want you at the table before I count to three. One . . ." If your child can tell time, you may even consider setting a timer so that he can see how much time he has before he needs to make the transition.

Depending on the age of your child, any of the following are appropriate strategies for reassuring your slow adapter:

- Talk to your child about the change and validate her feelings.

- Soothe your child with words or a hug or hold him.

- Ask your child what it is she needs to feel safer and more secure with the change in environment.

- Pair something familiar with the unfamiliar.

As with most traits, giving your slow adapter a sense of control will go a long way in reassuring the child that he or she is safe. If your child is outside playing before dinner, instead of just telling him to come in and eat, ask him first, "Would you like to throw the ball one more time before you come to dinner?" Another example of giving a sense of control is "I am trying a new peanut butter. Would you like raspberry or strawberry jam on your PB&J?"

6. Approach or Withdrawal

This temperament focuses on a child's initial reaction to new situations, new ideas, or strange people, places, or things (including food). Does your child approach a new food willingly or back away from it and yell "No!" before even giving it a chance?

This trait is usually connected to adaptability, as a child who is slow to approach a new food is also usually slow to adapt to a new food. The difference between the two is that the temperament of approach/withdrawal is your child's initial response to a change while adaptability is how your child adapts over time to the change.

1 **How does your child first react to a new food?**

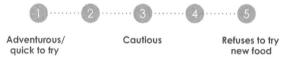

Adventurous/   Cautious   Refuses to try
quick to try   new food

2 **Do your children get upset or fussy when a new food is presented?**

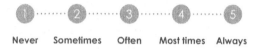

Never   Sometimes   Often   Most times   Always

3 **Does your child get upset with surprises—for example, he thinks he's having chicken for dinner but at the last moment you made pasta?**

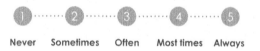

Never   Sometimes   Often   Most times   Always

4 **When eating at a new restaurant or with new people, does your child have a hard time eating because she is very shy and withdrawn in the situation?**

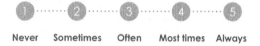

Never   Sometimes   Often   Most times   Always

Just because your shy child immediately reacts negatively to a new food does not necessarily mean that he or she does not like it.

If your child scored between 4 and 6, he or she is quick to approach new situations and food. These are usually the adventurous eaters who are a pleasure to cook for, as they will eat mostly anything or at least try it first before saying that they do not like it. A score of 14 or higher means you have a slow-to-approach child who will try a new food after much work and with multiple exposures and a lot of encouragement.

Strategies to Help the Slow Approacher

It helps to realize that these shy eaters are just expressing a biological trait and cannot help being anxious about trying a new food. Just because your shy child immediately reacts negatively to a new food does not necessarily mean that he or she does not like it. Some children are just more hesitant to try new foods than others. You can learn to work with your shy eater, but don't expect your shy/slow-to-approach child to try a new food without effort.

A slow-to-approach child takes a long time to warm up to new people, situations, and food. Understanding that your child has no control over his or her initial reaction will help you to keep your frustration in check. There is nothing that you can do to make your child jump in and eat a new food or not be shy when meeting a new person. Having a shy child means that you add the extra time he or she needs to warm up to your daily routine. Being steady and consistent wins the race with the shy child.

Continue to introduce your child to a new food over and over again. As you learned previously, a child can take ten to fifteen attempts before liking a new food. The shy child will be on the high end of this range.

Preparing shy children is essential. The following strategies will help shy children to get ready to try a new food:

- Let your shy child know beforehand that you will be serving a new food at breakfast, snack time, lunch, or dinner. He will have time to prepare instead of being surprised with a strange food on his plate.

- It helps to ask your child to think about what she wants to say before just reacting negatively when something new is set in front of her. Teach her to take one deep breath first before she makes an assessment when given a new food to try. This deep breath will help to calm and center the child who easily rejects new food.

- Ask your shy child to help you buy the new food, wash or prepare it, and serve it on his plate. This exposure helps him become familiar with the new food before he is expected to eat it.

- Keep the conversation casual and matter-of-fact. You do not want to make a big deal about your expectations, as this will only serve to make your child more resistant.

- Do not introduce a new food if there have been other changes in your child's environment. Like the slow-to-adapt child, shy children can usually only handle one change at a time.

Encourage your shy child to try new things. It will help if you view your child's interaction with a new food as similar to her meeting new people. She does not know this food, so you would take the same steps that you would when introducing her to a new person. As much as you wouldn't make her go up and hug a stranger, you also would not expect a shy child to take a bite of a new food the first time she "met" it. She needs to touch it, smell it, and lick it first.

Create a reward chart with a finger, nose, and mouth. Add a sticker each time the child touches, smells, and then tastes a new food. Your goal with a withdrawn child is to get him to try that first bite, which may be all it takes to get over the fear of the initial taste. Now if your child is also a sensitive child, you need to take baby steps to increase the number of bites slowly over time, too. If your child is not sensitive, then he may just eat the rest of his meal easily after the first bite.

Your goal with a shy child is that of cheerleader, "I know you will like this chicken once you try it." The worst thing you can do is to react when your slow approacher reacts negatively. If you respond with an equally charged frustrated exclamation of "Just eat it!", then your withdrawn child will just dig in her heels harder, and there is little to no chance that you will get her to eat her meal. If this does happen, apologize: "Sorry, mommy is really tired. I know you don't want to try the chicken, but I bet if you take one bite you will change your mind."

On the flip side of cheerleading is letting your children know that you understand that they are fearful of trying a new food: "I know you are uncomfortable about trying the broccoli, but I know you can do it. Remember how much you like carrots now but were afraid to try them at first, too?"

7. Persistence

This temperament is also referred to as frustration tolerance because it concerns your child's ability to concentrate or stay on task despite frustration. Can your child concentrate and finish a project, or does he give up easily when he becomes frustrated, bored, or tired with what he is doing? A child who sticks with a task despite distractions, frustration, and boredom is very persistent. One who gives up easily is considered easily frustrated. As children age, they develop more of a tolerance for activities, so your very young child may be able to handle more frustration as he ages. Find out whether your child is persistent or easily frustrated when it comes to eating and shopping.

1 **In general, does your child become easily frustrated when working on a task?**

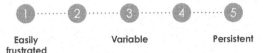

Easily frustrated   Variable   Persistent

2 **When your child wants something at the grocery store, does she take no for an answer or does she persist?**

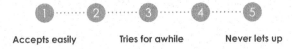

Accepts easily   Tries for awhile   Never lets up

3 **When your child doesn't like what is served for meal or snack, does he accept it easily or persist until he gets what he wants?**

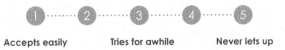

Accepts easily   Tries for awhile   Never lets up

4 **Does your young child get easily frustrated when feeding herself? For example, how does she react if the eggs keep slipping off of the fork, or she can't get enough soup on her spoon? Does your older child get easily frustrated when following a recipe or preparing a meal?**

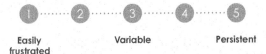

Easily frustrated   Variable   Persistent

If your children scored a 6 or lower, they are easily frustrated and have a hard time staying on task. A score of 18 or higher puts your children in the very persistent category. Read how to work with your persistent or easily frustrated child below.

Strategies to Deal with a Very Persistent Eater

If you give in to the demands of a persistent child and buy that candy or let him have hot dogs again for dinner, then you are just teaching him to keep asking until you give in. The persistent child is basically learning that you have a breaking point, and giving in just serves to make him try harder the next time.

Say no to the persistent child's demands, remain firm, and discuss future possibilities if he behaves: "You cannot have that candy bar now." If he asks again, say, "You can have a candy bar for your daily treat after you eat your lunch." If he asks yet again, say, "If you ask one more time, you will no longer be allowed your candy bar for a treat today." And then follow through with this statement if need be.

Children who are very persistent will also have a hard time stopping their current activity to come to dinner. They are so engrossed in playing, reading, or doing a project that they may lose track of time and not even realize that they are hungry. If this describes your child, give him ten-, five-, and one-minute warnings: ten minutes before you expect him to come to a meal, touch him on the shoulder and give a ten-minute warning; five minutes before dinner, do the same thing; and at one minute before, go over to your child and gently steer him away from his activity to the table or the bathroom to wash up.

Keep to a schedule because your persistent child may very well never stop what he is doing to eat.

Many times, a persistent child does not hear you because he is so involved in what he is doing. You may think that your child has trouble hearing or that he is ignoring you. This is not usually the case; most likely your child has gone to another place in his head, and the best way to break in is to touch him lightly. Screaming is not effective and will only serve to jar and frighten your persistent child. Remain calm so that you do not engage in power struggles.

Also, keep to a schedule because your persistent child may very well never stop what he is doing to eat. Creating regular mealtimes, eating at the table, and letting him know beforehand that a meal is almost ready are all great steps to take to prepare him for eating throughout the day.

Strategies to Help an Easily Frustrated Eater

Children who get easily frustrated will give up at the slightest indication of "this isn't fun anymore." They may start eating with gusto and then get bored easily and want to leave the table. Easily frustrated children have a hard time sitting still, not from an activity standpoint, but from a boredom perspective.

You would use the same strategies with an easily frustrated child at the table as you would for an active one: Start small and work your way up to having your child stay seated for the entire meal. Setting small realistic goals is key. Start with three bites before allowing a short break and work your way up to an entire meal for the young child. For an older child, set a timer for five minutes with three-minute breaks and increase the time slowly until he or she can sit through a meal.

Easily frustrated children are the ones who pitch a fit when the milk comes out of the bottle too fast or too slow. They are also those children who give up quickly when learning to use a spoon, fork, and cup. You may find yourself still spoon-feeding your three- or four-year-old because he does not like to do it himself. As tempting as it is to give in and feed your young child, resist and encourage him instead to feed himself. He will get better at it if you don't always do it for him.

After a long day, it can be very frustrating to have your child whine for you to feed him. If possible, take turns with another adult in encouraging your young child at the table. If your child refuses to feed himself when you know he can, then excuse him from the table until he is ready to eat by himself. Start with small, realistic goals—tell your child, "Serve yourself three bites of food and then you can be excused for a minute"—and continue increasing the number of bites until he is feeding himself.

If watching your child struggle is difficult for you, look the other way. Some parents, especially if they have a hard time with messes or are quick at picking up new skills themselves, have little to no patience for their slow learner. If this describes you, give yourself a time-out at the table if you cannot look away or disguise your discomfort.

As a last resort, allow your easily frustrated child to bring one thing to the table. Make sure it is small, does not require a battery or plug, and doesn't make noise so that it doesn't interfere with anyone else's mealtime. Allow your child this "privilege" as long as he continues to eat. If he does not, remove his item from the table. Your goal is to use this bribe to train your easily frustrated child to be able to sit for the entire meal. Once he accomplishes that, you can remove the toy or activity. To engage the child who is easily bored, you may also consider having everyone tell a story, play word games, or just talk about their day in a fun and engaging manner.

8. Regularity

When it comes to children's biological functions (sleep, hunger, and bowel movements), they can either have a set schedule every day, or they can be unpredictable when it comes to these biological functions. In terms of food, children who tend to get hungry and eat at the same time each day are considered regular, and those children who do not follow a schedule or predictable pattern are considered irregular. Determine where your child is on this continuum by answering the following questions.

1 **Would you consider your child's biological functions (hunger, sleep, and bowel habits) to be predictable each day?**

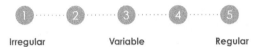

Irregular   Variable   Regular

2 **Does your child have a bowel movement every day around the same time?**

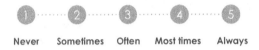

Never   Sometimes   Often   Most times   Always

3 **Does your child get hungry around the same time each day?**

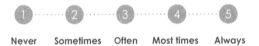

Never   Sometimes   Often   Most times   Always

4 **In general, does your child need to eat meals at the same time each day?**

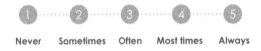

Never   Sometimes   Often   Most times   Always

You may or may not be able to answer these questions easily or at all. For the baby and young toddler, it may be easier to assess their daily routine because so much of it revolves around feeding and eating.

If you were not able to answer the questions on the quiz with certainty, do the following to determine your child's regularity temperament: Take some time to observe your child to see whether she actually follows a schedule. This will mean that you need to let up on your routine a bit to see what her natural routine is throughout the day. If you have an older child who tends to stick to a regular schedule for sleep, chances are she will tend to get hungry at the same times every day, too. Observe your child for three to four days to see whether there is a pattern to her hunger and eating schedule.

The important part of regularity is determining whether your child has a regular cycle and if so, whether you are meeting her needs as they arise. For instance, I have met a lot of parents who have a rough time with their child not being hungry at dinnertime because he has eaten a huge snack at 4:30 p.m. When they observed their child's hunger schedule they realized that their son was ready to eat dinner at 4:30 or 5 p.m. each day, and by not serving dinner until 7 p.m., they were stressing their child and thus themselves when the crying and whining and demanding started at 4:30 p.m.

Many parents try to hold back their child's hunger by filling them with snacks because in their mind, 5 p.m. seems too early to eat dinner or it is not convenient or even possible for them to have dinner ready this early each night. The following advice will help you learn to work with your child's eating and hunger schedule.

Strategies to Help Eaters with Regular Schedules

You have children who follow a regular schedule if they scored a 14 or more on the quiz questions. For these children, matching their need with your ability is key. Parenting a child who is regular can be a dream as long as it fits with your schedule; otherwise, it can be a challenge. For instance, for the child who needs to eat dinner at 5 p.m., what do you do if you are at work at that time? What do you do if your child is not hungry in the morning but needs to catch the bus? You do the best you can do in these situations.

For the child who needs to eat dinner earlier, make enough for dinner the night before so that there are plenty of leftovers. Your child can eat the reheated dinner from last night at 5 p.m. instead of eating a snack at this time. When the rest of the family sits down to eat dinner later, your child can have a smaller portion if he is hungry. Either way, have your child join everyone at the table.

Make sure that your children do not go longer than three hours (closer to two if they are three years or younger) without eating regardless of whether they are regular. The amount they eat at each meal or snack will depend on their hunger cycle. If you discover that your child is very hungry at 10:30 every morning and you need to fuss with them at breakfast, lower your expectations at breakfast and concentrate on a larger healthy snack at 10:30. A glass of milk or a protein drink with a piece of whole grain toast can serve as a breakfast, and a substantial midmorning snack can consist of fruit and half a sandwich.

The goal for children with irregular routines is to try and get them on some sort of regular schedule that allows for enough flexibility for fluctuations in their appetite.

Strategies to Help Eaters Without Routine Schedules

If your child does not seem to have a regular routine, it will be more difficult to assess whether he is eating the appropriate amount of nutrients and calories. Children with irregular hunger cycles may eat a lot one day and little the next. Most children have some days when they eat a lot and some days when they eat very little; children with irregular temperaments, however, live this way most of the time. As long as your children are consuming a diet in which 90 percent of it is made of whole foods (fruits, vegetables, healthy protein sources, and whole grains), then you have little to worry about because they will be able to listen to their internal message of satiety (I am full).

More likely, picky eaters with irregular schedules eat a lot more processed food high in salt, solid fat, and added sugar. In this case, you need to set a clear goal for what you will allow from this junk-food category. Let your children know that:

- They can have one treat a day.

- They must eat their healthy food before their treat.

- They may have only one juice a day.

- The rest of the time, they can choose from low-fat dairy, whole grains, healthy protein sources, and fruit and vegetable options.

You cannot let children, especially those with irregular schedules, have total control over what they eat, as they will almost certainly choose unhealthy food and beverages most of the time.

The goal for children with irregular routines is to try and get them on some sort of regular schedule that allows for enough flexibility for fluctuations in their appetite. You want to serve your child with an irregular schedule three meals a day and adjust the serving size according to how hungry he is. Encourage him to eat a little something (a whole grain, vegetable, and healthy protein source) at mealtimes, but if he is truly not hungry, have him join everyone at the table anyway with the understanding that this meal will be served again when he is actually hungry. This way the "irregular schedule" child will not use this temperament to get out of eating meals to focus just on snacks.

You can fill in the gaps and work around your child's unpredictable schedule with snacks; just make sure that they are healthy. You may even see after a while that your child's appetite will adjust to a more regular routine once he or she gets used to eating breakfast, lunch, and dinner at the same time each day.

9. Quality of Mood

This temperament reflects your child's predominant mood: For instance, is he or she usually happy or unhappy? Is your child's disposition one that is usually cheerful and sunny or glum and negative? Children are born into this world optimistic and positive, pessimistic and negative, or somewhere in between. You may already know exactly where your child falls on this scale, but if you have any doubt, take the quiz below.

1 **In general, where does your child rate on this quality of mood scale most of the time?**

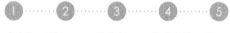

Pessimistic   Gloomy   Variable   Optimistic   Happy

2 **Will your child readily and with enthusiasm try new foods, or does she usually have a negative attitude about trying a new food or recipe?**

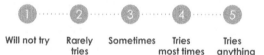

Will not try   Rarely tries   Sometimes   Tries most times   Tries anything

3 **When your child sits down to a meal, does he usually have something negative to say about the meal before even giving it a try?**

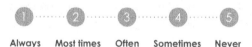

Always   Most times   Often   Sometimes   Never

4 **When grocery shopping or planning meals, does your child usually say something negative, such as "You never let me get what I want," "You never cook something I like," or "You always make Billy something he likes but you never do that for me"?**

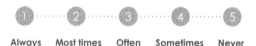

Always   Most times   Often   Sometimes   Never

This temperament looks at the general tone of your child's behavior and responses. Is your child easygoing and happy or fussy and unhappy around food most of the time? Lucky for you, if your child scored an 18 or higher, you have a delightful, easy-to-please child at the table. If, however, your child scored an 8 or below, then you most likely want to pull your hair out at mealtimes. It is especially hard for parents who have a sunny disposition to understand and not take personally their child's fussy and unhappy disposition. Read the suggestions for feeding a negative or pessimistic eater below.

Strategies to Help the Negative Eater

When dealing with a child who has a more negative outlook on life, it is important to know that you did not do something wrong to make him this way. Your child was born with his mood and disposition. The best thing that you can do is to accept your child the way he is and stop trying to please him at every turn in hopes that you will make him happy. If you use your child's mood as a barometer, you will be chasing the wind. Stop trying so hard to change a child who sees the world through negative glasses. Once you do that, you have won half the battle. If, however, your normally happy child turns negative and moody, you will want to look into that further.

It helps if you do not take your child's negativity at face value. If she expresses her displeasure when you serve her a meal, take a deep breath and tell yourself that she is just reacting negatively because that is what she is hardwired to do. Think of her reaction in a humorous way to tone down the situation. For example, see your child as a quacking duck whose response is just a "quack" before the meal.

The following strategies will help you to work with your negative eater:

- Hear what your negative eater has to say.

- Ask him to take a long deep breath with you to interrupt his initial negative response.

- Encourage him to start eating.

- If your child is easily distractible, use that to your advantage as well.

Here is an example: You have just served dinner when Mary says that she is not going to eat it. You say, "Let's take a deep breath together." Then breathe in for a count of four and breathe out for a count of four loudly so your child can follow your lead. "I know you said that you do not want to eat dinner. That is too bad because I know you will like it if you try it, but that is your choice."

If she still won't eat, try to distract her. "Look here, I served your favorite potatoes." Once she begins eating she may decide to eat the broccoli that she protested about at the beginning of the meal. If neither of these examples work, take it up a level. "If you really won't take a bite, you may be excused and go to your room, but remember that when you are hungry, this is what I am going to serve you."

Eating Out with the Negative Eater

When a child who is usually negative has an angry outburst or says something inappropriate in public, the worst thing you can do is throw gasoline on the fire by getting angry and yelling back. Instead follow these steps:

- After the outburst, ask your child to take a couple of deep breaths together with you. Exaggerate your in and out breaths so that the child can follow your breathing pattern.

- Remove the child to a private area.

- Get down to her level so that you are face-to-face and hold her hands in yours.

- Look your child in the eye and let her know that you heard what she said by repeating it back to her and teach her why what she said was not appropriate—for example, "I heard you say that the pasta looks disgusting, but that is not appropriate. You hurt the cook's feelings."

- Give the child an alternative so that she can learn how to express her negative feelings in a more acceptable way: "We cannot say that a food is disgusting, but you can say that you do not like how it looks or that you prefer to eat something else."

- Ask the child to explain in more depth why she did not like the food. For all you know, she did not like the parsley garnish, which would be an easy thing to fix.

- Let her know that she can return to the table after she apologizes for her inappropriate words: "I am sorry that I said the pasta looked disgusting." Do not ask her to say something that she does not believe. For instance, you would not ask her to go back and say that the pasta did not look disgusting.

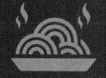

CHAPTER 6

Five Eating Personalities—How to Help Your Child Eat Healthfully

In this chapter, I have made it easier for you to deal with your picky eater in a fun and engaging way by describing eating personalities and characters who show up to dinner.

There are five main categories of eating personalities, each containing its own characters. The five categories are as follows:

1 Easygoing Eaters

2 Anxious Eaters

3 Strong-Willed Eaters

4 Distracted Eaters

5 Tasters

You will learn about each of these five groups of eating personalities along with a detailed description of the characters that fall under each group. Once you read through the five main categories that follow, you can jump to the characters that you recognize. But do not stop when you find one personality that matches your child, as most picky eaters have multiple eating personalities.

1. The Easygoing Eater

This type of eater is easy to feed because you do not need to spend time coaxing and encouraging the child to take a bite or finish the meal. These eaters will try most new foods without too much fuss. Issues with these eaters arise when they are misunderstood or when they eat too quickly and without much thought to what they are doing. When children eat too quickly, their stomachs do not have time to tell their brains they are full, which can lead to taking in too many calories at one sitting.

Not many children are healthy, Easygoing Eaters who eat mindfully, slowly, and without fuss. You can enjoy watching these Easygoing Eaters, but do not blame yourself if your child is not one of them. You did not create your child's temperament deliberately; your genetic makeup may have had something to do with your child's temperament, but that was not in your control.

The following characters fall within the Easygoing Eater category:

- **The Grazer** is an easygoing eater who needs her calories spread out throughout the day and has trouble eating large meals at one sitting. If you try and limit snacks with the grazer, give her too much junk food, or force her to eat a large meal, she will not do well.

- **The Gobbler**, on the other hand, eats with speed and without reservation. This type of easygoing eater usually takes in too many calories, so it is important to watch how much he eats.

2. The Anxious Eater

Some children are born afraid to meet new people or try new experiences while others are eager to jump right in. Anxious Eaters are the former; these children resist trying new foods and spend a lot of time and effort keeping their eating episodes similar and predictable. Anxious Eaters like to control their eating experiences, and that usually means that they eat the same thing day after day. Because of this, their diets are limited in variety.

The characters who are anxious or fearful around food are the following:

- **The *Neophyte*** resists trying any new food or drink.

- **The *Toucher*** will not eat a food that has touched another food.

- **The *Inspector*** spends a lot of time pulling apart a meal to see what is in there before he or she will begin to eat.

3. The Strong-Willed Eater

When most of us think about picky eaters, we imagine stubborn eaters who refuse to eat anything that they do not want. These Strong-Willed Eaters will go to extreme lengths to get the food that they want and will refuse to eat any food they do not feel like eating. Parenting a Strong-Willed Eater is difficult for most parents because it takes a lot of energy and patience to parent effectively. The following characters fall within this category:

- **The *Short Order Diner*** will ask for a separate dinner from the one you just prepared. He will ask either for one of his favorite meals or the opt-out option you have at home, usually a PB&J sandwich.

- **The *Snacker*** is the child you often find rummaging around your kitchen cupboards or freezer right before dinner. The Snacker picks at her meals and eats the majority of her calories after meals in the form of prepackaged snacks. This character usually has a diet high in sugar, salt, and unhealthy fats and low in produce.

- ***Dr. Jekyll/Mr. Hyde*** says that he loves a food one day only to refuse to eat it the next. This eating personality has a favorite food that he focuses on for days, weeks, and even months only to announce that he no longer likes it.

- **The *Actor*** gags or acts up when you serve a food she does not like, but if anyone else served it she would eat it without issue.

4. The Distracted Eater

Some children are intensely focused when they eat, but others often wander off—in mind and in body—to other things. The Distracted Eater has a hard time focusing on one thing for any length of time. These eaters are easily swayed by electronics, pets, siblings, and plenty of other stimuli at the table. Getting a Distracted Eater to focus long enough at mealtime can be challenging for many parents. The following are characters of Distracted Eaters:

- **The *Talker*** sits down to a meal and half an hour later, has barely touched her plate because she has been so busy talking. The *Talker* is so occupied that she does not pay attention to the hunger cues in her body or the sights and smells of the food in front of her. She has a hard time turning off her chatter long enough to eat, or she just plain forgets to eat her meal.

- **The *Player***, who can be either active or sedentary, would rather play than do anything else. The active *Player* has a hard time calming his body down and cannot sit still comfortably long enough to be able to eat his meal. The sedentary player is highly focused and intense; making it hard to drag him away from whatever he is doing to eat.

5. The Taster

This group of eaters is led by their taste buds. It is thought that 25 percent of children are what are called supertasters. When these children taste something bitter, they sense it as being *extremely* bitter. A sour taste that may not register in one child may be too much for the supertaster. Although many children are led by their taste buds to prefer processed foods, the characters that fall into this group are *ruled* by their taste receptors. The following are Tasters:

- **Mr./Miss Bland** will only eat food that has limited and similar tastes. They are the ones who eat a lot of white, processed foods, such as bread, crackers, and plain macaroni.

- **The *Dipper*** will not eat unless his food is dipped in a sauce.

- **The *Junk-Food Junkie*** is a prisoner to his preference for sweet or salty foods and beverages.

- **The *Drinker*** wants to drink her meals and avoid chewing. She would rather fill up on milk, juice, or soda and call it a day. This eating personality starts very young and can linger throughout childhood if not attended to.

Begin Here

You learned all about feeding practices in chapter 2: which to avoid (emotional feeding), which to always encourage (mirroring, teaching nutrition to kids, providing support and access to healthy food), and which need to be set according to your child's individual needs (monitoring, controlling, restricting foods, and "eat then treat").

For each of the following descriptions of eating personalities and characters, remember the positive feeding practices you learned earlier, and you will be directed as to how much monitoring or control you need to exert as well as when it is necessary to be stricter regarding treats and using food as a reward.

1. The Easygoing Eater

The *Grazer*

Temperament: Active, regular schedule, and distractible

Overview: Prefers to eat smaller meals more often

Diet quality: Can be healthy or unhealthy, depending on the quality and amount of food served at each sitting

Tommy eats small amounts of food all day long. When mealtime comes, he eats a small portion and an hour or two later is looking for more. He is constantly hungry and often asks for something to eat between meals. He gets very cranky and acts out if too much time goes by without eating. You are worried because you think he should be eating more at mealtimes and snacking less. You may also be concerned that he is eating too much in general.

Grazers love to eat smaller meals throughout the day instead of sitting down to eat a large portion for breakfast, lunch, and dinner. They most often have a hard time sitting for extended periods of time and are easily distracted. They are very much like *Players* in this aspect. *Grazers* can also be easily distracted in general and flit from activity to activity throughout the day. When mealtime comes, they eat breakfast, lunch, and dinner as long as it doesn't take too long.

Grazers are regular in the sense that they usually need to eat every two hours or so. Their mood seems to be closely linked to how often they eat. It is not unusual to see a meltdown, even in an older child, if more than two hours pass without having something to eat.

Grazers need snacks between meals, but not too many—they need to be hungry enough to eat their meals at mealtime. Many times Grazers are misunderstood and fed too much or allowed to eat mostly processed junk food at snack time. Once you determine that your child needs to eat more frequently, you can be better equipped to avoid his mood swings by giving him wholesome, healthy food every couple of hours. Too much junk food will only aggravate a Grazer.

Being a Grazer is natural for the small child. Younger children's stomachs are smaller, about the size of their fists, so they are not able to eat as much as older children. As such, they need snacks between meals to get all the nutrients they need to grow healthy and strong. This way of eating is actually very healthy as long as your child is eating a variety of healthy whole foods in appropriate portions. Your Grazer will be able to regulate how much she needs to eat throughout the day as long as processed treats are not allowed more than once a day. If your Grazer does not eat a healthy diet, check out the other eating personalities to see what else may be going on.

With some children the constant need for food may also indicate an issue with blood sugar control. Children who have trouble regulating their blood sugar levels need to eat frequently to prevent wild swings in blood sugar levels. Behaviors you will often see in children with blood sugar issues include shakiness, acting out, impulse-control problems, and zoning out, especially between meals and after eating candy or other sugar-laden foods and beverages. Get your child checked out if you feel that his blood sugar issues may be contributing to your Grazer's need to graze, especially if what he wants to graze on are sugary items.

Strategies for the Grazer

Grazing is actually a healthy eating behavior if done properly. Eating smaller, more frequent meals throughout the day will help small children get all the calories and nutrients they need, and it will help all children maintain better control over their blood sugar levels if they are sensitive to sugar. As long as Grazers are getting the required amount of calories and nutrients that they need from healthy options, there is no need for concern. If, however, your Grazer is undereating or overeating, especially on foods high in solid fats and sugar (junk food), then you need to intervene. Your Grazer may be a Junk-Food Junkie, Mr./Miss Bland, or a Neophyte as well.

Grazers with sugar issues will often seek out foods and beverages that spike their blood sugar levels, and because of this, they tend to eat more sugar than they should. If you are concerned that your child is eating too much or too little, check it out by determining how many calories and nutrients your child consumes on a daily basis. You can do this by writing down everything your child eats for a minimum of two days and as many as seven days.

Have the diet records analyzed by a professional nutritionist or dietician, or you can analyze them yourself by using the tools online at the USDA's My Pyramid Tracker (www.supertracker.usda.gov). After you enter the diet records, the tool will compute a detailed analysis of your child's diet. From this feedback, you can determine whether your child's diet provides the right amount of calories and nutrients or if adjustments need to be made.

The most important thing that you can do for your Grazer is to make healthy food and beverage options available to her throughout the day, especially midmorning, midafternoon, and between dinner and bedtime (if dinner is eaten early). Keep water along with cut-up fresh fruits and vegetables and some protein (e.g., cheese sticks, chick peas) accessible in an easy-to-reach place. Having access to healthy options is essential for the Grazer and will prevent potential crashes in blood sugar from occurring, especially if protein is available.

As long as weight is not an issue and the options are all healthy, you need not worry about your Grazer's frequent eating; just make sure she does not eat so much at snack time that she eats nothing for dinner. The key to feeding the Grazer is to understand that this is the way your child needs to eat, so it is best to be prepared by having healthy food available. This is not a behavior to turn around or push through. Everyone's body has its own needs, and respecting this is crucial for long-term health. If you suspect a blood sugar issue, follow up with your child's pediatrician.

You will need to lower your expectations for the Grazer at the dinner table. Because she has been eating smaller meals throughout the day, don't expect her to eat as much as someone who has not snacked and grazed throughout the day. You still want to make sure that there are two hours between snacks and mealtime, though.

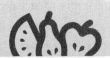

SUMMARY OF STRATEGIES FOR THE GRAZER

- Feed your *Grazer* smaller, more frequent meals; do not let more than two to three hours pass between eating episodes.

- Make sure you stop snacking two hours before lunch or dinner.

- Make healthy food and beverage options available throughout the day.

- Lower your expectation of how much the *Grazer* needs to eat at mealtimes.

- Limit treats to one a day.

- Monitor your child's food intake for a couple of days to make sure your *Grazer* is getting the right amount of nutrients.

The *Gobbler*

Temperament: Intense, not focused when eating, persistent

Overview: Eats meals or desserts very fast

Diet quality: Can be healthy or unhealthy depending on the quality of food served; tends to overeat

You are serving dinner and before you can put everyone's plate on the table, Jennie has finished her dinner and is asking for dessert. No matter what is for dinner, Jennie eats it up quickly, kind of like she has a train to catch.

When you watch *Gobblers* eat, they pick up their spoon or fork and they don't look up until they are done. It is hard to have a conversation with *Gobblers* during a meal because their mouths are full and they don't like to be interrupted.

There are two types of *Gobblers*. The first is a delight to feed because he or she will eat anything that is served. You will, however, need to work on having this type of *Gobbler* slow down because eating too fast is not healthy. The other one, the picky *Gobbler*, eats only certain foods, mostly junk food and dessert. This sort of *Gobbler* is actually a *Junk-Food Junkie* who eats way too fast. These children have real issues with sugar and may even have an addiction to junk food. *Junk-Food Junkies* get very upset when they don't have the food they crave. They overindulge when it is available and usually have some sort of meltdown afterward because of the sugar crash. All of these aspects are similar to what alcohol or drug addicts go through. If this sounds more like your child, jump to the *Junk-Food Junkie* (page 169).

The *Gobbler* is the one who will eat most anything, but when he does, he tends to overeat because he eats too fast. This type of eater does not give his body the time it needs to process that his stomach is full (usually twenty minutes). Some children gobble and go because they are in a rush, but the *Gobbler* eats this way all the time. On the one hand, he seems extremely focused, as he is so intent on the act of eating that he tunes out everything else. On the other hand, he is disconnected to his body. The *Gobbler* does not seem to even be conscious of chewing, tasting, and appreciating food.

Make sure that your child is not eating fast because she is stressed or anxious. If this is the case, work with your *Gobbler* to lessen her anxiety while using the following strategies to get her to slow down.

Strategies for the *Gobbler*

The best strategies for *Gobblers* are portion control, getting them to slow down, and practicing mindfulness. This personality knows what they want and desires it with intensity, and you can use this drive to your advantage. At the dinner table, make sure that your *Gobbler* eats all the healthy food first: vegetables, then protein, and last, carbohydrates. That way she can fill up on the fiber in vegetables, which will help to limit her ability to overdo it with the carbohydrates or protein.

Always offer age-appropriate portion sizes (see chapter 4), even when eating out. If your *Gobbler* is served a huge portion at a restaurant, ask for a box immediately and place half the meal in it. Say to your *Gobbler*: "Wow, this portion is huge. Let's box up some of this delicious food to go so that you can have it at home tomorrow."

If your *Gobbler* still wants more food after he has eaten an adequate portion, make sure twenty minutes have gone by before saying yes. Teach your *Gobbler* what appropriate serving sizes are as he ages. *Gobblers* cannot trust their bodies to say "stop" because they are eating too quickly, so they need to focus on external stimuli, such as serving sizes, to do that.

Your job with *Gobblers* is to teach them how to work with their propensity to eat fast and with abandon. Getting your *Gobbler* to slow down will take time and effort. If your *Gobbler* eats her entire meal in five to ten minutes, she has a good chance of overeating. Strategies that you can use to help your *Gobbler* slow down include:

- Serving different components of the meal separately, at times that are spaced out.

- Have your *Gobbler* put his fork down between bites.

- Try to engage your *Gobbler* in conversation.

- Gently remind your *Gobbler* to slow down, knowing that she has difficulty doing so.

Finally, know that your *Gobbler* is born with an intense and persistent temperament, and there is little that you can do to change that. You may consider trying some sort of mindfulness or meditative practice with your child. Teaching her how to use her breath to slow down is a great way to give your *Gobbler* control without drawing undue attention at the table. Learning how to use breath control will also help your *Gobbler* in other areas of her life.

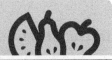

SUMMARY OF STRATEGIES FOR THE *GOBBLER*

- Teach your *Gobbler* what appropriate serving sizes are.

- Slow down mealtimes using the strategies listed in this section.

- Train your child, or find someone who can teach your child, to use breathing technique to slow down.

- Make sure twenty minutes have elapsed before serving seconds.

2. The Anxious Eater

The *Neophyte*

Temperament: Sensitive, intense, and slow to approach

Overview: Fearful about trying new foods

Diet quality: Usually very limited and high in unhealthy nutrients (sugar, solid fat, and salt) and low in healthy nutrients (vitamins, phytonutrients, and fiber)

Every time you offer Bobby a new food, he screws up his face, yells "yuck!", and pushes his plate away. He hasn't even tried it yet, but there is no budging him, no matter how much you coax. His diet is very limited, because he will eat only familiar foods. You are scared because you don't want to force him, but you know this limited diet cannot be healthy for him.

We are all born with some degree of neophobia (fear of the unknown) surrounding food. There is an evolutionary explanation: When we started to toddle around and explore our environment, not all food was edible. Some foods were poisonous, which tended to be bitter-tasting, and others were healthy. Because of this, we learned to be wary of trying new foods. This leftover survival instinct is difficult to work with in the current food environment in which bitter-tasting foods (vegetables) are the healthy items and the sweet foods are usually unhealthy.

Children come into the world with varying degrees of fear when presented with a new food, and there are times in children's lives when this fear heightens and wanes. The degree of neophobia that is being referred to with the *Neophyte* is one that limits the child's diet to the point that he will eat only ten or fifteen foods. A diet that is this restrictive cannot supply all the nutrients a growing child needs.

Although some children may outgrow neophobia, if left unattended, it can continue to progress to a point where your tween or teenager eats only a very limited diet. There is also new evidence to suggest that it may continue into adulthood. Adults who eat only a few foods are said to have a selective eating disorder, and this type of disorder may soon be added to the new psychiatric diagnostic manual.

The *Neophyte* is high on the withdrawal scale and needs a lot of coaxing and extra time to get used to a new food before being asked to try it. You will never get a *Neophyte* to try a new food the first time you plunk it down in front of him or her unless you make a lot of effort or offer a huge bribe. A child who may or may not like a new food is definitely not a *Neophyte*. *Neophytes* are very intense about their feelings of not wanting to try a new food or drink.

Strategies for the *Neophyte*

Fearing new food is something that is developmentally appropriate and embedded in your child's genetic makeup. Accepting that your child was born this way will help to lessen your stress level. Knowing you did nothing wrong to create a child who is fearful of new foods and to understand that it is actually a natural impulse will give you the insight and patience you need to stick with your *Neophyte* when he or she tries new foods.

If you wait for your *Neophyte* to try a new food on his or her own, it may never happen. This child is the definition of a child with a slow to approach or shy temperament. You would want to use all the strategies described in the previous chapter:

- Lower your expectations of how quickly your child will accept a new food.

- Do not push a shy child to try new things; instead, follow her lead.

- Give your child permission to take his time to get to know a new food.

- Be a cheerleader encouraging new things while at the same time acknowledging your child's fear.

- Prepare your slow to approach child by letting her know what is coming next.

- Get him involved in buying, preparing, and serving the new food.

- Focus on getting your child to take that first bite.

- Introduce one new food at a time when there have been no changes in your child's environment.

- Serve her favorite food with a new food at mealtime.

A new food is scary to *Neophytes*, so they will resist trying it, say they do not like it before they have tried it, and do anything in their power to avoid eating it. It is vital that you encourage your child to try new foods that they are resistant to and work cautiously with those foods they visibly fear. All children need to be nudged along the path to making healthy food choices, as it is not an innate impulse anymore. The *Neophtye* just needs a stronger and longer nudge.

Make sure that you encourage, not force, your child to try new things and remember that it can take up to a dozen attempts before your child will like a new food enough to eat it. If your child shakes or cries when approached with a new food and you have tried to get her to touch or smell it, stop what you are doing and seek professional guidance.

Take the example of a child I worked with who was so afraid of fruit that she visibly shook if I walked into the room with an apple or orange. If I told you that this four-year-old went from fearing fruit to eating two new fruits in a thirty-day period would you believe me? Well, she did, and this is how: I made a sticker chart and bought her favorite stickers. On the chart were three columns. One column had a picture of a finger, one had a nose, and the other had a mouth. Her first challenge was to touch a fruit at the grocery store that she wanted to work with. Once she was comfortable touching that fruit, she began smelling the fruit. After being comfortable with smelling the new fruit, she was asked to take one lick. The lick turned into one bite, then two bites until she learned to like the fruit.

The key to this exercise is to let the child be in control: Tell the child what to expect with each baby step, never push her beyond her limit, reward her with a sticker or points for each positive step she makes, and move on to the next step when she is ready.

Neophytes investigate new food like a detective at a crime scene. Give them the space to feel, taste, and even play with it a little. The young child and baby naturally play with their food, whereas the older child can "play" by picking out a new food at the store, coming up with a recipe, and helping to prepare it in the kitchen. Keep offering children food that they initially don't care for in small serving sizes, which you can increase over time.

Remember to "play" with foods that are in the "I don't love it, but I also don't hate it" range discussed in chapter 1.

Control is essential for kids in most situations and especially regarding food. The trick as a parent is to give them the illusion of control until they mature enough to be able to handle the issue themselves. When introducing babies to a new food, place the food on a fork or spoon but stop before you reach their mouth. Let them come in for a bite instead of forcing it into their mouths or else it won't be successful and both of you will end up frustrated. With older children, give them a choice between two healthy options so that they feel in control as well: "Do you want green beans or carrots with chicken for dinner?"

Involve your older children in the selection and preparation of a new food. Have them select the produce at the market and teach them how to tell whether it is fresh. At home, they can wash and, depending on their age, cut up the new food during dinner preparation.

If your child takes one look at the new food and exclaims that he hates it or finds it disgusting before trying it, respond by saying, "You cannot say you do not like it before you have tried it yet." Consider it the "no-thank-you bite": The child has to take one bite, but if he does not like it he can say "No, thank you" to another bite. The next time around he has to take two bites, and so on until he is eating a appropriate serving. If you have already given your child time to get to know the new food, then encourage him to take one bite. The one-bite rule and the "eat then treat" statements are going to be your most powerful tools for broadening your Neophyte's palate.

For the extremely resistant child, use the reward point system to get her to take that first bite. It is the first bite that *Neophytes* are most afraid of. If you can distract them or provide an amazing incentive, they will be able to focus on the reward and not the new food. Once they have tried the first bite, they can now determine from their own experience just how good or bad the taste was. Continue with the point system until your child is actually eating an appropriate serving size of the food without you having to work hard at it. When your child has succeeded in eating an entire serving of the new food a half dozen times, you can stop the reward system.

In the future, your *Neophyte* may continue to resist the new food, and that would signal that he or she may have the temperament of a slow adapter. If your *Neophyte* is slow to accept new food, you can always respond by saying, "That's too bad because that is what is for dinner. Tomorrow night you can pick the vegetable, but tonight it is broccoli that you have learned to eat (or like)." Keep your comments short and sweet and move on to eating the meal.

Last, remember that an extremely resistent *Neophyte* may actually be a child with an undiagnosed sensory issue. Perhaps your son or daughter is just reacting strongly to a certain color, taste, temperature, or texture of new food. Refer to the previous chapter for tips on how to distinguish whether your child has a sensitivity issue before implementing these strategies if you have any doubts.

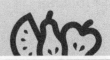

SUMMARY OF STRATEGIES FOR THE *NEOPHYTE*

- Use the one-bite rule and increase the amount of a new food your child must eat by one bite each time you serve it.

- Don't fall for or allow "Yuck" to stop you from serving your *Neophyte* the new food over and over again.

- Give your child a sense of control by letting him pick the vegetable that will be served with dinner.

- Let the *Neophyte* play with her food so she gets to know it first.

- Remain patient and continue to have your child try the new food twelve to fifteen times—that's how many times it can take before your child will tolerate the new taste.

- Use the "eat-then-treat" rule: "If you eat your green beans, you can have dessert."

- For the very resistant *Neophyte*, use the point-reward system for motivation.

- Serve your child's favorite food with the new food on his plate.

The *Toucher*

Temperament: Sensitive, intense, easily frustrated

Overview: Does not like when one food touches another food

Diet quality: Usually limited in variety and amount

Jimmy is sitting at the table eating his dinner when he screams. You think something horrible has happened—and to him something horrible did happen. His peas rolled into his mashed potatoes and his dinner is ruined!

Touchers are very picky when it comes to how they want food served on their plate. They may or may not be picky when it comes to the foods they like, but they certainly have a need to control the way their food is organized on the dish.

Also, *Touchers* often have a prescribed order in which they eat foods. Heaven forbid the chicken touched the carrots or the broccoli collided with the mashed potatoes. Events like these can lead to a complete meltdown, and parents find themselves trying to sort out the collision. To a *Toucher*, however, once one food has touched another, there is no going back. The foods are ruined.

The *Toucher* does not understand why you don't already know that the carrots need to be kept separated from the rice, for instance. He usually feels very misunderstood and frustrated because to him his response is normal. Your *Toucher* is probably expressing a sensitivity issue whereby he does not like it when two textures, tastes, or colors are combined.

If your child's negative response is not sensitivity driven, then your *Toucher* has a high need for control. Once you understand this, you can let your guard down and stop fighting her on what you may consider a silly issue. This is certainly a time when you want to give in to your child's demands, as it is futile to fight with your child on this issue. You may not completely understand why your *Toucher* needs it this way, but knowing that this is essential will help you have an easier time working with her on this issue.

Strategies for the *Toucher*

It is easier to accommodate *Touchers* than it is to change their behavior. Relatively speaking, this is an easy personality to please. These children tend to be very determined and strong-willed individuals, yet also easily frustrated and sensitive. They may or may not need to control other aspects of their lives, but when it comes to food, a perfectly cooked, delicious meal would be ruined by one chance encounter of peas bumping into potatoes.

Sit down with your *Toucher* to talk about his needs when it comes to serving food. Depending on the age of your child, you may gain some very important insights; maybe he just doesn't like when certain foods touch but doesn't mind when others do, for example. Let your *Toucher* know that you will be happy to accommodate his needs as long as he can let you know the specifics.

Purchase plates with dividers for the *Toucher*. These plates will save many meals from being ruined by preventing a comingling of foods. You can find both strong disposable plates as well as permanent varieties. It is also a good idea to give your child some control in this situation as the *Toucher* is likely one who needs to feel in control a lot. Have her serve herself, and if she is too young to do this effectively, you can help her guide the serving spoon.

Another trick when feeding a *Toucher* is to serve her one item at a time. Start with the food that is the healthiest—usually the vegetable—and when she is done with that serve the rest of the meal one item at a time. You can ask her which one she prefers next, the entrée or side dish. If eating food in a predetermined order is important to her, give her a say in what is served next.

The good news is that most *Touchers* will eventually outgrow their need to keep their food separate. If you think about it, you probably haven't seen many tweens or teens doing this.

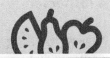

SUMMARY OF STRATEGIES FOR THE *TOUCHER*

- Have a conversation with your child to understand the specifics of how she wants her meals and snacks served.

- Once one food has touched another, serve a new plate, as there is no undoing the comingling of food.

- Control is essential for the *Toucher*; get his feedback as to how things need to go for her at the table.

- Give in to your child's demands and serve her food on a plate that has dividers.

- As soon as your child is old enough, have him serve himself.

The *Inspector*

Temperament: Pessimistic, slow to approach, easily frustrated

Overview: Suspicious about eating foods, distrustful, anxious to find something wrong with their food

Diet quality: Usually a very limited diet

You serve dinner, and everyone has been eating for five minutes when you look over at Brenda. She is busy turning over her chicken breast and picking apart the rice. Her head is so close to the food you fear she may fall in. You would smile and think that she would make a good surgeon with the precision with which she is dissecting her meal if you weren't too tired after a long day to assure her yet again that everything is perfectly fine with her food.

Inspectors would make good detectives; they are usually suspicious of all new things and people. When meeting a new person, *Inspectors* will take a long time to warm up and say hello. They do the same with food that is put down in front of them, whether it is a new food or an old standby.

My older sister wouldn't eat anything until she dissected it with the meticulousness of a neurosurgeon, and I am sorry to say that to this day she still does this. She is forever pulling food apart and asking what everything is: A green parsley fleck on her piece of chicken could be the end of the meal for her. In all her years of inspecting, it actually served her well only twice, which reinforced and perpetuated this behavior.

Inspectors have a strong desire to know everything, and it is difficult to be sneaky with them around. They are very curious and may have an issue with trust in general, which may also manifest itself around food. For *Inspectors*, I don't suggest using the technique of hiding healthy food in food your child will eat with ease. If you are caught just once, eating meals will become very difficult and they will likely not be able to trust you again. Following are effective strategies for working with an *Inspector*.

Strategies for the *Inspector*

Inspectors are another eating personality, like *Touchers*, who do really well if you give in to their basic need of having to know what they are eating before they will eat it. Because they are distrustful, persistent, and pessimistic, *Inspectors* can be difficult to handle at the table. Start by realizing that no matter what you do, you will not be able to stop your *Inspector* from examining her food. What you can do is accept that this is a strong innate need and allow her to engage in a limited amount of inspecting as long as she does not affect others around her with her comments.

If this behavior is setting off other siblings at the table, ask the *Inspector* to dissect his meal in the kitchen before joining the others. Let him know that while seated at the table, negative comments are not allowed. You need to teach your child that this behavior makes it difficult for others to eat their meal. If your *Inspector* gets very upset and needs to say something, excuse him from the table so both of you can talk about it in the kitchen. Do not allow this private conversation to occur more than once a meal. It may also be necessary to limit your *Inspector*'s questions to one or two at mealtime because this behavior can get out of hand with your child refusing to eat the majority of the food on his plate.

A reward chart will also help to lessen the amount of negative outbursts or inappropriate comments. If neither of these strategies works, excuse your *Inspector* from the meal for a time-out with these instructions: "We do not talk negatively about our food at the table. I have looked it over and it is perfectly fine; if you cannot sit here and eat your meal without complaining, you need to go to your room for a time-out. When you are ready to eat your meal without complaining, you may come back to the table to eat with the rest of the family." It is best to allow time for inspection, but it is not all right for a child to comment negatively once everyone is sitting down eating. For more advice, refer to food rule #6 in chapter 3: No "yuck" is allowed at the table (page 73).

As with the *Neophyte*, the *Inspector* has a hard time with new foods because they are foreign to her. Use lots of encouragement and give your *Inspector* plenty of time to get used to a new food; she will need more exposures to learn to like a new food than most other eating personalities will. Give her the opportunity to get to know what she is eating using the same techniques described in the *Neophyte* section: touching, smelling, and tasting, for example.

One of the best strategies for *Inspectors* is to get them involved in the cooking and preparation of their meal. This way they know exactly what went into the food they will be eating and will be less likely to pull it apart. Have a younger child in the kitchen while you prepare the meal and talk through what you are doing. You can even have her wash the herbs or produce before adding it to the dish. If at all possible, you do not want your *Inspector* to see her meal for the first time at the table.

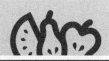

SUMMARY OF STRATEGIES FOR THE *INSPECTOR*

- Never hide food in your *Inspector*'s meals or snacks.
- Let your child play with his food: touch, smell, and lick it.
- Get your *Inspector* in the kitchen to help prepare her meal or snack.
- Allow inspecting to be done in the kitchen before coming to the table or limit the amount of inspecting allowed at the table.
- Do not allow negative comments at the table. Excuse yourself and your *Inspector* to the kitchen for a chat. Limit these chats to one per meal.
- Allow him enough time to get used to a new food.

3. The Strong-Willed Eater

The *Short Order Diner*

Temperament: Intense, persistent, focused, slow to approach

Overview: Doesn't eat what is served; insists on a separate meal at mealtime

Diet quality: Usually a very limited diet

You rush home from work and throw together a delicious meal. Before you can eat a bite, Billy takes one look at his meal, pushes his plate away, and yells that he wants chicken nuggets instead. You tell him no and to eat his meal. Five minutes later Billy is not giving in so you figure it is easier to make the darn chicken nuggets. You grab a glass of wine and head for the kitchen. Before you know it, you are making a separate meal for Billy five out of seven nights of the week.

Short Order Diners are exhausting busy parents everywhere. No matter what is served for dinner, this child wants something else. This eating personality is used to getting his way and is pretty intense, strong-minded, and persistent about getting what he wants. A *Short Order Diner* is not easily distracted and has a hard time accepting new foods.

For many parents, this type of eating personality is not hard to accommodate at first, but before you know it, things have gotten out of hand. It usually starts with good intentions at a young age, usually after babies transition to table food. What was once an easy task of opening jars of baby food turns into creating a separate meal for your toddler and then your young child. Soon your baby is six years old and you are still making a separate meal so she will eat it. Parents with multiple children have it even harder as they sometimes end up making a different meal or variations of a meal for as many children as they have.

No parents like to see their child upset and many think it is easier to give in than to put up a fight. It is difficult, especially after a busy day, not to give in to your *Short Order Diner*'s request, especially if she screams and cries to get her way. Letting children have whatever they want all the time, however, sends the wrong message and puts children in the driver's seat when they are too young to know how to make healthy or informed decisions. Children do not have the intellectual capacity or the desire to make healthy choices, so parents have to help make these decisions for them. At the end of the day, the time you save by giving in is not worth the price your *Short Order Diner* has to pay later on with his or her health.

Short Order Diners are similar to *Mr./Miss Blands* in that they both usually have limited variety in their diets because they choose the same small handful of favorites time and time again—chicken nuggets, mac 'n' cheese, and hot dogs are all typical choices. This type of diet will provide nowhere near the nutrition that kids need to fight disease and remain healthy.

Strategies for the *Short Order Diner*

The transition between baby food and table food is one of the most important transitions in a child's life. The *Short Order Diner* is most often created during this transition. Most babies love fruits and vegetables pureed at home or from a jar. Your job as a parent is to continue to foster that appreciation of these important foods, and you do this by continuing to offer such foods to them often, even—and especially—when they don't seem to like them anymore.

After transitioning from baby food to table food, offer your toddler the food that the rest of the family is eating but in age-appropriate portions cut up in small pieces. By feeding children the same food as the rest of the family, they get used to the fact that they must eat what everyone else is eating. If you don't start offering them a choice and say no when they ask for alternatives, then they will quickly learn that there is no other option. They will stop, or never start, demanding a separate meal. If you are serving a new food, make sure your children take at least one bite the first time, two the second time, and so on until they are eating a serving.

For established *Short Order Diners*, simply do not offer to make another meal. When they ask for something different, first ask them to try the meal you have prepared and enforce the one-bite rule. If that doesn't work and they continue to demand another meal option, let them know that they have two choices: They can eat the meal you prepared or leave the table. When and if your *Short Order Diner* announces that he is hungry later on that night, continue to offer him the same dinner, reheated, of course.

Your *Short Order Diner* will eat when he is hungry enough, unless of course he has a physical or emotional issue that precludes him from making this decision. Remain firm, with a smile on your face, because once your *Short Order Diner* knows that you are serious, he will finally understand that he must eat this dinner. Caving in will only cause your *Short Order Diner* to be more persistent. If you are offering a new food or dish, lower your expectations as to the amount of food you expect your *Short Order Diner* to ingest. As long as he tries the new food, he can fill up on the rest of the meal.

You are not being a bad parent by encouraging your child to eat the dinner that you prepared. Many parents of *Short Order Diners* are either super-busy and don't have the energy to fight the nightly battle with these eaters or they are indulgent parents who have trouble saying no. Limits and rules are important for all the behaviors that you are teaching your child, and eating is no different. As a parent, you have the long-term vision for your child's health in mind. You need to make healthy decisions for your child until she is old enough, smart enough, and able to do it herself.

Many parents allow children to choose one standby that their kids can go to if they don't like a meal. This is usually cereal or PB&J sandwiches. There are several problems with using standbys. It doesn't teach variety, and usually the options are processed foods that are high in sugar and low in fiber. Having an opt-out meal also teaches children that they do not have to eat the healthy stuff if they do not want to.

If you do choose to have an opt-out standby, make sure it is a healthy option. Each option should include a vegetable. That way your children will learn that they need to eat a vegetable at every meal so they don't use the opt-out approach to avoid eating their veggies. Some healthy options include hummus on whole grain bread with cucumber or tomato slices or sunflower seed or nut butter on whole grain tortillas with cut-up veggie sticks.

Make the opt-out option available no more than once a week. You and your child can keep track of it with a chart on the refrigerator. If your child currently eats her opt-out meal many nights of the week, reduce the number of nights you allow it by one night a week. *Short Order Diners* do better with gradual changes.

Sometimes the *Short Order Diner* is just looking for another way to have control over an ever-changing world. Encourage your *Short Order Diner* to take part in some aspect of the meal no matter what his age is; he can do some sort of food preparation, choose the night's vegetable, or any other task that acquaints him with what is being served. If you involve your child in selecting and preparing the food, he comes to the table knowing what is for dinner and will be less likely to be surprised and announce that he won't eat the meal and demand an alternative. Let him have some input when selecting the menu ("Should we have broccoli or carrots with the chicken?"), and you may even give him one night a week when he decides what to eat—within healthy parameters, of course.

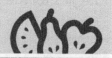

SUMMARY OF STRATEGIES FOR THE *SHORT ORDER DINER*

- Transition toddlers to the family meal by offering them what everyone else is eating, pureed at first and then cut into tiny pieces.

- Enforce the one-bite rule.

- Do not make another meal and instead keep offering the child the meal you prepared or excuse her from the table until she is hungry enough to eat it.

- Avoid or limit opt-out options to no more than once a week and make sure the opt-out is a healthy option.

- Let your child know beforehand what his next meal will be.

- Involve your child in meal preparation so she is not surprised with what is served.

The *Snacker*

Temperament: Intense, persistent, regular

Overview: Prefers to fill up on snacks and pick at meals

Diet quality: Usually unhealthy and most often made up of highly processed food and little to no produce

About an hour or so before mealtime, Luke is rummaging through the cabinets for a snack. You tell him to wait and not fill up on junk but he screams that he is starving. He shows up to dinner, takes a couple of bites, and says he is full. Within 10 minutes, he is back looking in the refrigerator for dessert and continues to snack for the next several hours filling up on processed food.

A *Snacker* may at first sound like a *Grazer*, but the essential difference is that a *Snacker* will resist eating mostly healthy food while the *Grazer*'s diet is made up of many healthy options: the former is a strong-willed eater while the latter is an easy going eater. The *Snacker* can be seen as a merging of the *Grazer* and the *Junk Food Junkie* in that he wants to eat foods high in salt and sugar and resists fruits, vegetables, whole grains, and meals in general. If it comes pre-packaged, or even better, in a single serving container, he is all for it and gobbles that down.

This character is born out of a parent's fear that if a child says that he is full, you must believe him without question. The *Snacker* figures this out quickly and uses it to his advantage to let his taste buds lead the way to what he desires or craves. Many times these desires may appear to be fine on the outside, but if you look at the amount of sodium, processed grain, solid fat and sugar that are in the foods the *Snacker* goes for most often, you would be surprised.

This is a typical post-diner snack for the *Snacker*: she took several bites, announced she was full, and then proceeded to consume chocolate milk, gummy fruit snacks, a cereal bar, yogurt, and a single serving package of cookies. *Snackers* will get the calories that should have been consumed at dinner through their snack choices, plus an extra 74 grams of sugar, which equals about 2¾ cups of added sugar a week or 140 cups of added sugar a year! It's not looking so good now, is it?

If you looked at the nutritional quality of their diet, they do not fare any better than the *Junk Food Junkie*. While they may not be asking for cookies, cakes, and candies, they are asking for gummy fruit snacks, breakfast cereal, pudding, granola bars, and sweetened yogurt, which are highly sweetened foods just the same. For many parents, yogurt with 15 to 20 grams of added sugar per serving or pudding with 15 grams of added sugar may seem like a healthier choice than a chocolate candy bar that has similar amounts of added sugar. The *Snacker* is looking for the sweet and salty taste of processed food just like the *Junk Food Junkie* but doing it in a more subtle way. Once you understand that this is your child's motivation, look at the Nutrition Facts labels to see how much sugar and salt is in the snacks your child is asking for. If it is not a healthy choice for snack time, replace it with fruit, vegetables, whole grains, and healthy protein options.

Strategies for the *Snacker*

The *Snacker* is just a character who has developed bad eating habits, and with any unhealthful habit, reversing it is the cure. That may be easier said than done, but by following the strategies below and remaining firm, you will turn the *Snacker* around in no time. If you are an indulgent or lenient parent, reversing this bad habit may be harder for you than it is for your *Snacker*. By now you know why it is important to be firm while taking your child's needs into consideration at the table as well as why it is so important that your *Snacker* eats his meals, too.

Snacks should be looked upon as a way to get your child's healthy diet requirements met and not as a sugary and salty free-for-all. Begin turning around your *Snacker* by setting realistic goals at the table. Refer to chapter 4 for serving sizes and Appendix B for the amount of food your child needs to consume every day. Once you are clear on what your child should eat during the day and at mealtime, then you can let your *Snacker* know just how much you expect him to eat before he is allowed a snack. You will need to use the *eat then treat* rule often as well as exert a high degree of monitoring and control until you have turned this unhealthy eating habit around.

You may even consider creating a visual to help your Snacker understand what is expected. Purchase marbles, poker chips, or stickers in at least five colors that represent a serving size of food at mealtime. For example, one green chip represents one vegetable serving, one red chip one protein serving, one yellow chip one whole grain serving, one blue chip one fruit serving, one white chip one glass of milk or dairy alternative, and one black chip one treat. Count out, by referring to Appendix B, how many of each of these chips you need; divide them into meal and snack time and place them in baggies (each baggie representing a snack or meal); when your child eats a serving, she puts that chip into a bowl, and by day's end, all the chips should be used up.

When you begin to turn your *Snacker*'s eating habits around, sit down with him and explain what you will be doing. Let him know that until he eats his meal he will not be able to have a snack; that the meal will be presented again the next time he is hungry. He should also be aware that snacks will not be allowed within 2 hours of a meal. Have set meal times so that he knows he cannot eat a snack after 4 p.m. if dinner is at 6 p.m. You want your *Snacker* good and hungry by the time dinner is served. A hungry *Snacker* is more willing to eat his meal whereas a full *Snacker* will just pick at it.

When your *Snacker* announces that she is starving within the two-hour window of mealtime, allow vegetables or fruit only during this time. The reason for this is twofold; it will call your child's bluff if she was just trying to get a treat, plus these healthy options will add to her daily nutritional requirement, not take away from it. Cut-up vegetable sticks dipped in hummus and fruit slices with nut butter are all healthy options that go toward meeting your child's daily fruit and vegetable requirement. You child can grow and thrive just fine without processed snacks; she cannot do either though unless she gets her requirements for fruits, vegetables, protein, and whole grains every day.

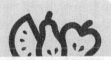

SUMMARY OF STRATEGIES FOR THE *SNACKER*

- Create realistic expectations at meal time.
- Do not offer snacks or dessert until the meal is eaten.
- Limit the amount of snacking that is allowed.
- Make sure a fruit or vegetable is eaten at every snack.
- Set the rule that snacks are not allowed within 2 hours of mealtime.

Dr. Jekyll/Mr. Hyde

Temperament: Can be any mixture of temperaments

Overview: Likes a food one day and hates it the next

Diet quality: Usually limited in variety

Penny has been eating broccoli and salmon for months now and just last week she said it was yummy. Today, however, she announces that she hates it and won't touch another bite.

Children learn how to eat and what they like and dislike throughout their childhood. There are two categories of children who like food one day and hate it the next: Children with a normal variance in their diet and children who overeat a food to the point whereby they never want to eat that particular food again.

Most kids at one point or another during childhood will say that they don't like a food that they have liked in the past. This is completely normal behavior. Everyone has days when they just do not feel like eating something that they have eaten before. This occasional resistance to food previously liked is not considered picky eating per se; rather, it becomes an issue when children resist previously liked foods often or cut a food out of their diet completely.

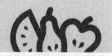

KEEP SERVING THOSE SUPERFOODS

My son loved broccoli and salmon; I would serve this meal once a week and he gobbled it up every time. One night when he was five years old, he announced that he didn't like salmon or broccoli.

Instead of removing his plate and offering him another dinner, I turned to him and with a smile on my face said, "You may not like it but it likes you," and "You need to eat it." He looked at me with surprise and then went on to finish his dinner. He tried this three more times, and each time I repeated the same thing. He finally learned that this didn't work.

When he got older, around age six or seven, I taught him about superfoods, such as broccoli and salmon, and explained that these foods were so good for our bodies that we needed to eat them regularly. At age ten, he eats his broccoli with the understanding that it is not his favorite vegetable, but he needs to eat it because of the supernutrients broccoli provides.

My job is done. I am sending my child out into the world with the understanding that he may not love certain vegetables (or other healthy foods), but that doesn't mean he gets out of eating them.

At the table, *Dr. Jekyll/Mr. Hydes* tend to change their mind often, even during one mealtime. This type of eater can range from being quite independent and persistent to shy and distracted, but what many *Dr. Jekyll/Mr. Hydes* usually have in common is their limited diet. If a child has a lot of variety in his or her diet, eliminating several foods is not a problem, but with the child whose diet is extremely limited to begin with, removing one or two foods is a huge deal. A child with a limited diet is also at an increased risk of eating a food too frequently. These eaters latch onto only a handful of foods and eat them so frequently that they then get sick of a food and then it is gone forever.

Children will eliminate a food from their diet if they got sick after eating it (called taste aversion) or if they ate it so much that they got sick of it. Outside of those situations, something else is often at work the other times a child says that he or she no longer likes a food. As you learned previously, "I don't like it" can mean everything from "I am bored" to "My peas touched my potatoes."

Often, children use mealtimes to express their independence and test how far they can push back on rules or expectations. The power structure within a family is on display during family meals, and the power struggle between older children and their parents isn't left at the door when dinner is served.

Strategies for *Dr. Jekyll/Mr. Hyde*

The best way to prevent *Dr. Jekyll/Mr. Hydes* from eliminating a food from their diet forever is to not serve the same food at every meal or the same items day after day for each breakfast, lunch, and dinner. With the limited variety that exists in the diet of your *Dr. Jekyll/Mr. Hyde*, make sure that you spread the foods that he or she will eat over the day so that you are serving a different breakfast, lunch, and dinner three days in a row before you introduce the same item again—so, for example, your child can have chicken nuggets at dinner every fourth day. If your *Dr. Jekyll/Mr. Hyde*'s diet is so limited that there is not enough food for variety during three consecutive days, use the strategies you learned about in the previous chapter for dealing with the approach or withdrawal temperament (page 120) to introduce new foods into your child's diet.

It is okay to continue to encourage, not force, your child to eat something that he announces he doesn't want to eat anymore. Before you do this, make sure that your child is not eating so much of that food that he is getting sick of it. If this is the case, back off and serve that food no more than once every four days.

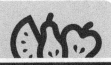

SUMMARY OF STRATEGIES FOR DR. JEKYLL/MR. HYDE

- Focus on making sure that your child does not eliminate a food forever from his or her diet.

- Do not serve foods that your child is stuck on too often.

- Broaden your child's diet to include enough variety for separate meals three days in a row.

- Encourage your child to eat the foods he or she does not like, especially if they are superfoods, and avoid the ones your child truly hates.

- Let your child know you heard what he had to say and encourage him to eat the food. Explain why he needs to eat it and serve it again once every four days.

The *Actor*

> **Temperament:** Intense, persistent, slow to adapt, slow to approach new food, probably sensitive
>
> **Overview:** Uses his or her acting skills to get out of eating an entire food group or many foods
>
> **Diet quality:** Usually limited in variety

Dennis's mission in life is to never eat a vegetable if he doesn't have to. When he eats with his mother, he gags every time he puts a bite of a vegetable in his mouth and his mom reacts with horror, immediately removing the offending food. However, when Dennis eats with his dad or at a friend's house, he will eat a vegetable with just one prompt. "Please eat your carrots" works just fine when mom is not around.

This is a true story: I watched my friend's child gag when she offered him any vegetable. He would look at his mother for a reaction, and as soon as he saw it, he knew he had won and didn't have to eat his vegetable. When mom was in the room he reacted negatively, but when she wasn't in the room he had no reaction. We did an experiment one day at my house where she didn't react when he gagged on the vegetable he was served. She remained calm and plastered a smile to her face while he made his noises. He kept looking at her to get a reaction and when he did not get the reaction he typically saw, he swallowed his vegetable. I don't know who was more surprised—the mother or the son.

This was very hard for my friend to do, as her natural reaction was one of protection. If you have a child who reacts negatively to many foods or one food group, you know how difficult this can be. Knowing when your child's reaction is real and when it is a

put-on to get out of eating something he does not like is essential when working with a child who gags when eating. Follow these steps to help you sort out if you are watching a play or a real issue with food:

1 First rule out any sensitivity issue or other physical or emotional disorder before deciding that your child is an *Actor*.

2 If your child avoids a single food group entirely (fruit, vegetables, grains, protein, dairy or dairy alternative) or a large number of foods, you need to work with her. If she just reacts to a small number of foods and her diet is healthy as a whole, then there is no need to intervene.

3 Experiment to see whether your child will eat a food that he normally reacts negatively to if you are not present. If your children will eat the food with ease when you are not around but gag when you are, there is a chance he is putting on a show just for you because he knows it will work.

4 Observe your child for a couple of days to see whether she reacts negatively only to healthy food and never to junk food.

Many misdiagnosed *Actors* have a sensitivity issue, which is why it is so essential to work with a professional who can rule this out before attempting to turn around a child who reacts negatively to many healthy foods or an entire food group. It may just be a texture issue, which may not seem obvious to you.

The biggest clue to look for is whether your child eats the offending food with ease when you are not around. If he or she does not, then your child likely has an undiagnosed sensitivity issue. In the absence of a food sensitivity issue, chances are you have an *Actor* at the table. *Actors* are very bright and learn early on that if they exaggerate their response to a food, mom or dad won't make them eat it, especially if they have a parent who is very sensitive and lenient.

When *Actors* eat a food they don't like or just prefer not to eat, they become quite dramatic and will make noises or go all out for the Academy Award by gagging. During this entire process, *Actors* are watching their parents closely to see whether they are achieving the desired effect.

Note that a very small percentage of children have an exaggerated gag reflex or severe textural disorders that can cause a gagging reaction. If your child has a developmental disorder, is autistic, or has a condition warranting medical intervention, then by all means seek expert advice for feeding strategies. It is always wise to err on the side of caution, especially when it comes to food and any sort of gag reflex. If you feel as if you are being played after ruling out any serious issue, then the following strategies may work for your little thespian.

Strategies for the *Actor*

The best strategy to use with the *Actor* is to keep a straight face and not react. This eating behavior is a dance whereby it takes two to tango. The child is dramatic and the parent feeds into the drama by reacting in fear and pulling back. It may be hard to not react at first, but try your best. Keep a smile on your face and remain calm. Children can pick up on their parents' vibes extremely efficiently.

If your child continues to react, say nothing and finish eating your meal. When you are done remove his or her plate without commenting and excuse your *Actor* from the table. This strategy will take time and usually doesn't work immediately. It may take many meals to change this behavior. If, after a month, you see no change, then seek out professional help if your child's diet is very limited.

You don't ever want to force your child to eat, but you do need to encourage eating, especially if he uses acting to get out of eating vegetables or any other healthy food group. The best technique for encouraging him to try a food that you really want him to eat because you know how healthy it is is to use the "eat then treat" technique: "If you eat your broccoli, then you can have dessert." You need to use something that is very motivating for the *Actor* for this to work; usually it takes the promise of some sort of prize or dessert to be successful. Once your *Actor* has gotten used to eating foods in a food group, then you can back off with the incentives.

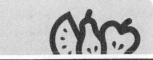

SUMMARY OF STRATEGIES FOR THE *ACTOR*

- First, rule out any physical or emotional issue that may cause your child to reject a food or food group.

- Do not react at the table when the *Actor* is putting on a show.

- Use "eat then treat" method to motivate your *Actor* to eat a food he or she does not like.

- Remove the incentive once your *Actor* can eat that food with ease.

4. The Distracted Eater

The *Talker*

> **Temperament:** Distracted and persistent
>
> **Overview:** Talks so much during mealtime the child does not eat enough
>
> **Diet quality:** Usually eats too little at mealtime

Molly sits down to eat but after a half hour she has barely touched her meal. She has been talking and talking throughout dinner. You are exhausted and tired of listening, but you don't want to crush her spirits. Secretly you just wish she would stop talking already. You must have asked her a dozen times to eat, but she doesn't seem to hear you. What are you supposed to do?

Mealtime is a great time to share stories about everyone's day, but if your child spends the whole time talking and doing very little eating, this is a problem. Your *Talker* usually doesn't eat enough at mealtimes and may or may not make up for it later. Your goal is to train your *Talker* to focus on his or her meal, give everyone a chance to speak, and leave the table after eating a sufficient amount of food.

The *Talker* does not seem to get when it is time to stop talking and give someone else a chance. Some *Talkers* are anxious and talk because they are nervous or uncomfortable while others are born being very social and approachable. If you have a child who is both, then you really have a *Talker* on your hands. *Talkers* are also easily distracted at the table, and all it takes for them to stop eating is for someone else to start talking.

Talkers tend to be very talkative elsewhere in their lives and learning when to speak and when to listen may be an ongoing struggle for them. If you already have effective strategies for managing a chatty child, then use these same strategies at the table. If not follow the suggestions here.

Strategies for the *Talker*

You want to determine whether your *Talker* is anxious at the table. If so, find out what is calming for your *Talker* and use that information to make her feel more relaxed. Your *Talker* may very likely be reacting to the chaos that is going on around her because she is easily distracted. Use the techniques described in chapter 4 for creating a calm eating environment for your *Talker*.

Teach your child how to transition from playtime to mealtime effectively. Just as the *Player* needs to run and jump before meals, make sure your *Talker* has had time to talk to you during his day before you sit down to dinner. If he did not, bring your child into the kitchen for talk time. Let your *Talker* know that you would love to catch up and that you can do that while the two of you prepare a meal. With this technique, not only do you give your *Talker* the necessary outlet to express himself, but you also get an opportunity to teach him how to cook and prepare food.

Let your *Talker* know that meals are an opportunity for everyone to share stories about their day, and if the *Talker* takes over the conversation, someone else at the table doesn't get a turn to share. If being quiet is difficult for your child, teach her a meditative or breathing technique whereby she learns to sit in silence without being uncomfortable. When everyone arrives to eat, give the child a gentle reminder before the meal: "I can't wait for everyone to have a turn to tell me about their day" or "Let's focus on our meal while we take turns sharing about our day."

Explain to your *Talker* that she can talk at the table as long as she continues to eat her meal. You may need to reach out and gently put your hand on your *Talker*'s arm to get her to focus on what you are telling her. Make this a "three-strikes-and-you-are-out" rule. If you need to remind your *Talker* more than three times to keep eating and stop talking, excuse her from the table until she can follow your instructions: "You need to have a break until you can learn that you need to eat while at the table. I love hearing what you have to say, but eating is what is most important right now." Pay attention to serving sizes so that you can accurately assess whether your *Talker* has eaten enough of her meal.

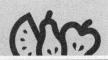

SUMMARY OF STRATEGIES FOR THE *TALKER*

- Rule out any anxiety issues in your child before proceeding.
- Create a calm eating environment to limit distractions.
- Teach your child how to sit in silence.
- Allow talking as long as eating is also occurring; three strikes and you are in a time-out.
- Have talk time in the kitchen while preparing meals together.
- Teach your *Talker* to give everyone a chance; have your child ask a question of someone else at the table.
- Focus on the transition time to the table: "Now is when we settle down and focus on eating."
- Place your hand gently on your child's arm to focus him.

The *Player*

> **Temperament:** Easily distracted, active, intense, focused, and persistent
>
> **Overview:** Has a hard time sitting still; would rather play than eat
>
> **Diet quality:** Varies depending on how much he or she eats at one sitting; tends to undereat at mealtime and fill up on snack foods with lower nutritional value later

Kyle loves to play; in fact, he would rather run around all day than eat. Kyle will come to the table only after his mom gets so frustrated that she threatens to send him to his room if he doesn't. Kyle takes two bites before he is off and running again. His brother Bryan loves to play Legos, and no amount of pleading with him will get him to the table to eat. He does not like to be interrupted and gets very upset when he is asked to stop playing to come to dinner, no matter how much warning he gets. Bryan will try to bring his Lego truck to the table to play. At the table, he will take one bite and jump off his chair to continue playing.

Having a *Player* in your house can be very trying, especially around mealtime. Whether you have an active *Player* who is always on the go, a sedentary *Player* who sits still and plays for hours, or a combination of the two, getting a *Player* to focus on eating is a challenge. You call your child for supper several times and have to resort to threats to get him to come and eat. Once your *Player* gets to the table, he can manage only a couple of bites before going back to playing.

Many parents have pulled their hair out because they do not understand their *Player*. Once you get that your *Player* is born with an active temperament and realize that she is not disobeying you by fidgeting, you are well on your way to working with your child. No amount of punishment is ever going to turn your active *Player* into a child who can sit still with ease. The active *Player* is easily distracted, especially if siblings are around.

The sedentary *Player*'s temperament is one that is high on focus and intensity. This type of child gets lost in what he is doing to the point that a party could be going on around him and he would not notice. Understanding that your sedentary *Player* is persistent and has an innate tendency to be superfocused will help you to realize that he is most likely not purposely ignoring you when you call him to the table. He just needs help to transition from one activity to another.

Your *Player* will not eat enough at mealtime if you do not help him to settle and focus. Resorting to snacks that are easy to grab and go is not a long-term solution for working with your *Player*. Instead, follow the strategies listed here for your active or sedentary *Player*.

Strategies for the Active *Player*

With the understanding that active *Players* need to move, create opportunities for them to do so without compromising mealtime or snack time. Make sure you allow your Player plenty of time to run, jump, and play before meals. For young children, break mealtime into bite episodes until you can train them to sit through the entire meal. Start with a three-bite minimum before being allowed a play break for two minutes. The play breaks are earned by eating three bites of food. If this goes well, the next day increase the number of bites required to earn a play break to four bites and continue this until your *Player* can sit through an entire meal.

For older children, you may want to use a timer and require them to sit for five minutes, take a three-minute break, come back for another five minutes, and so on. Slowly increase the time required to sit before a break until you have trained your *Player* to eat a meal without leaving the table. Refer back to the previous chapter and follow the strategies listed for the active child (see page 114).

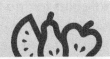

SUMMARY OF STRATEGIES FOR THE ACTIVE *PLAYER*

- Understand that your *Player* needs to move her body.

- Give your *Player* ample opportunity to get his energy out before mealtimes.

- Train your active *Player* to sit through a meal by slowly increasing her time at the table.

- Use play breaks as an incentive to get your *Player* to eat his meal.

Strategies for the Sedentary *Player*

Different strategies work for different ages of sedentary *Players*. For the young child learning to eat, distracting her with a toy on the highchair is fine as long as it is used only when needed. If it takes a toy to introduce a young child to a vegetable or to get him to sit still long enough to eat, use a toy now and again. At each meal, try to feed your child without a toy first. If he fusses too much, pull out a toy with the understanding that you will need to break this habit once your child is comfortable sitting still long enough to eat.

Once your sedentary *Player* can sit for a meal with ease, take the toy away at mealtime and use it instead as an incentive: "You can play with your truck once you finish your dinner." Tell your child, "Now that you are a big boy, you need to eat like mommy or daddy and that means that there is no playing with toys at the table." Your sedentary *Player* will adjust to this pretty quickly as long as you reward him with plenty of opportunity to play after eating.

For children older than two, refer back to the previous chapter and use the strategies listed for the focused and intense temperaments (pages 111 and 115). The strategies are also listed in the following summary.

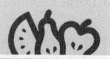

SUMMARY OF STRATEGIES FOR THE SEDENTARY *PLAYER*

- Remind your sedentary *Player* five minutes, three minutes, and one minute before mealtime that he needs to transition from playing to eating.

- Gently touch your focused child while she is playing to let her know she needs to stop playing in five minutes.

- Promise your sedentary *Player* that he can play once he eats his dinner.

- Let your sedentary *Player* know what you will be serving long before mealtime so she can process that information beforehand.

- Create a calming eating environment for your *Player*.

- Use a toy only briefly to introduce a new food or keep your young child at the table.

- Transition to using their toy as a reward for eating their meal.

5. The Taster

Mr./Miss Bland

Temperament: Sensitive, slow adapter, slow to approach, persistent

Overview: Eats only a handful of very bland foods

Diet quality: Very limited; lacking in fruits, vegetables, and fiber

You can count on two hands the only foods that Alice will eat, and they all seem to be white or beige in color. No matter what you cook for dinner, unless you serve chicken nuggets, mac 'n' cheese, or plain pasta with butter, Alice will not eat her meal. You have tried everything: adding sauces, hiding food in her mac 'n' cheese, but none of these strategies work. You can't believe that this kind of diet can be healthy for her and you are concerned.

Mr./Miss Bland has a lot in common with the *Neophyte* in that neither of these personalities will try new foods with ease. While the *Neophyte* eventually learns to like a new food, *Mr./Miss Bland* also has an issue with being a slow adapter and so takes a superlong time to learn to like a new food. Most parents do not have the patience for, or understanding of, how many exposures it takes *Mr./Miss Bland* to learn to like a new food and usually give up after only a few tries. When you put together a child who is slow to approach (resistant to new foods) and slow to adapt (takes a long time to get used to change), along with being persistent, you have a child who is very difficult to feed. You are correct in being concerned for your child's health with this limited diet.

Mr./Miss Bland's diet is most often devoid of one or more food groups, with vegetables, dairy, and fruit being the most common. This child tends to like processed carbohydrates (white bread, crackers, and pasta); few protein options (chicken nuggets and cheese); some fast food (French fries); and little to no vegetables. *Mr./Miss Bland*'s diet is so limited that it is deficient in essential nutrients. This eating behavior needs to be turned around because your child will most likely not outgrow this restricted eating pattern on his or her own.

It is likely that your *Mr./Miss Bland* is sensitive to tastes. When she tastes a slightly bitter or sour taste, she registers it as super bitter or sour. To test this out, give your child who is three years or older a little sip of tonic water (no more than 1 teaspoon) and watch her reaction. If I did this in a room full of people, some would spit it out because it tasted so bitter and the others would taste nothing. If your child has a strong reaction, then know that she is a supertaster for bitterness. All you need to do it put a little lemon juice in water to see how much sour taste your child can handle. Armed with this information, you will be better able to work with *Mr./Miss Bland*'s taste buds. Read on to add variety to your *Mr./Miss Bland*'s diet.

Strategies for *Mr./Miss Bland*

Understanding how your *Mr./Miss Bland* is hardwired is essential for reversing her unhealthy eating habits. Once you realize that it can take twelve to twenty exposures to a new food to budge *Mr./Miss Bland* into liking a new food, you will be better equipped to handle your child at the table. This information will lessen your stress and anxiety immediately because now you have a realistic timeline that works for your child who is slow to accept new foods into his or her diet. You may want to keep a chart handy to see how many exposures it takes your *Mr./Miss Bland* to like a new food. Like a science experiment, he or she may also find this very interesting.

If your child is supersensitive to bitter tastes often found in vegetables, salt will be your friend. Salt + bitter = sweet. Add a dash of soy sauce or a sprinkle of salt to broccoli, kale, collard greens, and other bitter-tasting vegetables to help your child tolerate the taste. You do not need to go overboard with the salt—a dash will do you. Over time, your *Mr./Miss Bland* will get better at tolerating bitter tastes, but he or she will always taste bitterness more strongly than someone who is not a supertaster. Play around with adding a bit of sweetness to things that are sour to see if your *Mr./Miss Bland* will like it better. The sweet doesn't get rid of the sour taste like salt does for bitter tastes; the sweet just competes with the sour on your child's taste buds to distract them.

Follow the Food Rules and do not allow your *Mr./Miss Bland* to say "yuck" at the table. Explain to your children that you do not expect them to like something the first time that you give it to them because it takes them time to learn to like a new food. Use this method for each new food you introduce, focusing on one new food at a time while pairing it with something your child will eat with ease:

- Have realistic expectations.

- Pair an unfamiliar food with a familiar food.

- Provide many exposures to a new food.

- Teach your child about himself.

- Introduce one new food at a time.

Here is how a conversation may sound with your *Mr./Miss Bland* when you serve her green beans for the first time along with the chicken nuggets she loves. If your *Mr./Miss Bland* reacts negatively to the green beans and refuses to eat them, say "I do not expect you to love these green beans, but I do expect you to try them. You will be seeing green beans quite a lot because I know it takes you some time to learn to like a new food." If your *Mr./Miss Bland* does not react negatively, then there is no need to say anything. For those who will not try even a bite, use *Mr./Miss Bland*'s favorite food as a way to entice her to take a bite using the same strategies listed for the *Neophtye* (the one-bite rule): "Once you try these green beans, you can have your chicken nuggets."

Finally, be aware that *Mr./Miss Bland* could have a sensitivity issue that prevents him from trying or liking many foods. Pay attention to the foods your child rejects. Are they a similar color, temperature, taste (spicy, salty, or sweet), or texture? If so, follow up with your child's pediatrician to rule out or confirm a sensory disorder.

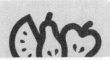

SUMMARY OF STRATEGIES FOR MR./MISS BLAND

- Set realistic expectations by understanding that your *Mr./Miss Bland* needs many exposures to like a new food.

- Check out sensitivity issues.

- Help your child to understand herself better at the table by counting how many exposures it takes to like a new food.

- Add salt to bitter foods and a dash of sweetness to sour foods to make them more palatable.

- Introduce one new food at a time and pair it with a familiar food on your child's plate.

- Use *Mr./Miss Bland*'s favorite food as an enticement to persuade them to keep trying a new food.

The *Dipper*

Temperament: Intense, usually a slow adapter, persistent

Overview: Will only eat foods dipped in a sauce, usually sweet/salty

Diet quality: Usually a very limited diet, high in sugar and/or salt

You served hamburgers and French fries with ketchup the night before, but tonight's menu is fish and broccoli. Little Larry screams for ketchup to dip his broccoli in. He refuses to take one bite until you put ketchup on his plate, and there it begins—a Dipper is born.

We all know that kids love to dip. Dipping is a tool that many parents use to get their children to eat food they may not necessarily like, such as vegetables and protein sources. Everything and anything seems to taste better when dipped in a sauce, not to mention the engaging fun factor of the dip. So what is the problem here? None, as long as your child eats food not dipped in sauce as well.

The *Dipper* is a child who has taken dipping to the extreme, to the point where he or she will not eat anything unless it is slathered in a sweet or salty sauce. The unhealthfulness of always needing to dip has to do with the following:

- The amount of sugar and salt that children consume by always dipping is most likely above their daily limit.

- Always hiding the taste of vegetables in dip or sauce prevents *Dippers* from learning to like the taste of vegetables. Their taste buds get used to sweet and salty tastes and want more of them, and they continue to dislike bitter-tasting foods like vegetables.

Determine whether your child is a healthy or unhealthy *Dipper* by answering these two questions:

1 Does your child need a dip to mask the taste of all foods?

2 Does your child use dips such as ketchup, BBQ sauce, soy sauce, steak sauces, sweet and sour sauce, honey, caramel sauce, and chocolate sauce on a daily basis?

If you answered yes to either question, then your child is an unhealthy *Dipper*. The sauces listed above should be occasional foods in your child's diet. Healthy, more frequent dip options include guacamole, hummus, and any dip made with plain low-fat yogurt, cream cheese, or sour cream and with limited added sugar or salt.

Take a look at the sugar and salt (sodium) content of ketchup and other sauces and notice how high these additives are in the list of ingredients. If sugar is one of the top three in a dip, then consider it a sweet that must be managed so that your child doesn't keep needing more and more of it. When it comes to more savory dips like cheese sauce, sour cream, or mayonnaise, use varieties low in fat and salt. It is always best, especially with younger children, to get them used to the taste of the vegetable plain so that they learn to like it before introducing dips.

Dipping is a learned trait. What starts off as the innocent addition of ketchup to fries can snowball for some children into the need to dip all their food, especially their vegetables. My niece is actually an extreme *Dipper*. She will not eat anything—and I mean anything—for breakfast, lunch, and dinner that she can't dip in ketchup or BBQ sauce. Like most unhealthy eating habits, this behavior is easy to teach and tough to break.

Both my sons have tried to add ketchup to everything including broccoli, beans, carrots, and sweet potatoes. It amazed me how quickly my one-and-a-half-year-old noticed his older brother dipping his food and asked for it himself. The first time I let him dip his fries into ketchup at dinner, he actually remembered it at breakfast and asked for ketchup on his eggs and toast. I drew the line quickly and said in a calm voice, "We use ketchup on only our burgers and fries and nothing else."

I am aware that I am teaching my sons eating habits for life, so I want them to understand why I am setting the limit. The toddler gets that "we don't do that" and the eleven-year-old can understand that he doesn't need the added sugar in the ketchup and that he needs to get used to the taste of vegetables, which the ketchup will mask.

You may think it is not a bad idea to let children dip their food in sauces as long as it gets them to eat their veggies. But what you are actually doing is training your child's taste buds to like and only eat foods with a sweet or savory/salty taste. Once you raise the bar from the natural sweetness of fruits and some vegetables to an artificial level by adding sugar, children will get used to that sweeter taste and then demand it at their next meal or snack. They will also seek out more sweet and salty tastes in their diet, which leads many to become *Junk-Food Junkies*. The good news is that once you reduce the sugar and salt in your *Dipper's* diet, your child will go back to eating low-sugar and low-salt foods once he goes through an adjustment period.

Strategies for the *Dipper*

If your child is dipping his food in sauces that are not high in sugar and salt, then there is nothing to fix, necessarily. Just make sure that your child will also eat vegetables without being slathered in dip. It becomes restrictive if there always has to be a sauce on hand. It also doesn't allow their taste buds to become accustomed to the basic taste of the pure food.

If your *Dipper* needs salty and sweet sauces to get anything healthy down, you will want to reverse this unhealthy habit. Slow and easy wins this race. This is one of those behaviors that first-time parents or extremely busy parents allow and then regret later on. When children start to eat table food, avoid adding sweet or salty sauces to their food. They don't need them, and without them, they will actually learn to prefer the natural taste of food.

Once children see their friends or siblings dipping, they will want to dip, too. It is best to limit the number of foods that you will allow to be dipped right away. What begins as "I need ketchup for my fries" easily turns to "Can I have ketchup for my broccoli, beans, etc.?" A great strategy is to use dipping in unhealthy sauces as a special treat that you allow no more than once or twice a week. Be creative and get your *Dipper* involved in coming up with some great recipes to prepare vegetables or protein sources. Some *Dippers* have a need for intense flavors; instead of using sauces loaded with unhealthy ingredients, use spices to provide the flavor they need. Some *Dippers* actually have a sensitivity issue and are using sweet sauces to hide the taste or color of food that they have trouble with. Do a taste test with your *Dipper* to find out whether he or she prefers strong flavors or more subtle ones.

Every day, feed your child vegetables without added sauces or strong flavors to train their taste buds to learn to like the taste of plain vegetables. You will most likely need to use the eat-then-treat rule to entice your child to eat carrots, celery, pepper sticks, broccoli, or cauliflower florets. Put these raw or lightly steamed veggie sticks out before dinner when your hungry child will eat anything.

Your child's taste preferences will develop based on the tastes of the foods you give him. If you get him used to green vegetables, he will like green vegetables. If you feed him fish, he will learn to like fish.

To reverse a *Dipper*, do so slowly. You need to set limits about which foods it is okay to have sauces and ketchup with, and then discuss these limits with your child. Eliminate ketchup from one food at a time, starting at breakfast and then working to lunch and finally dinner. Once she has made improvements, continue to enforce the limit on dipping as this behavior is easy to slide back into. In our house, ketchup is allowed on turkey burgers, homemade fries, and nitrate-free hot dogs, but I draw the line with vegetables.

If your *Dipper* still will not cooperate, take away the privilege of dipping. She does not get ketchup for her fries if she will not eat her vegetables, for example. Unhealthy dips are in the same category as treats because of the high salt and sugar content. As such, the eat-then-treat rule needs to be enforced. Once you understand that your *Dipper* wants her sugar or salt fix, you can begin to manage her appropriately by practicing tough love. Refer to the section on the *Junk-Food Junkie* if your child also eats a lot of sweet treats or junk food, as these two personalities often go together.

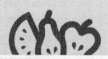

SUMMARY OF STRATEGIES FOR THE *DIPPER*

- Allow dipping with only a small handful of foods.
- At least once a day, have your child eat plain vegetables, raw or lightly cooked.
- Most dips are high in sugar and salt and should be used no more than once to twice a week.
- Reverse the dipping habit slowly by focusing on one meal at a time and one food at a time.
- Dipping is a privilege to be earned.

The *Junk-Food Junkie*

Temperament: Sensitive, intense, persistent

Overview: Will eat mostly processed junk food, especially sweetened foods and beverages

Diet quality: Usually a very limited diet high in salt, sugar, and saturated fats

For snack time, you are feeding Katherine salted crackers. No matter how many you give her she wants more and gets very agitated and a bit crazed the more she eats. She screams like her world is ending when you say no more; it never seems as if she is satisfied. Katherine usually comes to a meal filled up on snacks, says that she is full and can't eat another bite, but then screams for cookies and gummy fruit snacks within ten minutes of the table being cleared.

Children who are intense and persistent can be very challenging to manage, especially if you are easygoing and lenient. Even the strongest parents have difficulty with these two temperaments, particularly if they have little understanding of these innate tendencies. Even though your *Junk-Food Junkie* may have been born high on the intensity and persistence scale, a *Junk-Food Junkie* is only created when he or she is exposed to junk food. Most children left to their own devices will become a *Junk-Food Junkie* because processed junk food is super-tasty and is made to be addictive. Parents who are indulgent or hands-off usually have *Junk-Food Junkies* in the house.

The *Junk-Food Junkie* is an eating personality that a lot of us recognize. No sooner does he say he is full at dinner, he then asks for dessert or goes to the closet for cookies, chips, snack cake, or pudding. You may even recognize this eating personality in yourself.

Junk food is addictive and many children, not to mention adults, have a difficult time regulating how much they've eaten. A lot of us have seen a mild-mannered child turn into a screaming maniac over not being allowed junk food or being told they cannot have anymore. You know you have a *Junk-Food Junkie* if you are afraid of taking away your children's treat or saying no to him. This eating personality will let his feelings be known in no uncertain terms. *Junk-Food Junkies* crave, seek, and sneak junk and have withdrawals if not allowed it.

Many *Junk-Food Junkies* have an issue with sugar control. Over time this unhealthy eating habit will likely lead to diabetes or heart disease, so it is important to reverse the high daily intake of sugar, solid fat, and salt in your child's diet. When *Junk-Food Junkies* start the day with a sugar-filled breakfast of cereal, juice, and toast and jam or toaster cakes, the sugar level in their blood rises very quickly. Because what goes up must come down again, their blood sugar level will plummet, which will prompt them to reach for sugar to raise it again. This roller-coaster ride is not fun nor is it healthy for your child.

Low blood sugar doesn't feel good; children dealing with it get cranky, emotional, moody, and even shaky. Accepting that your child has a possible addiction or just plain cannot stop eating junk food will make it easier for you to understand and work with your *Junk-Food Junkie*. Follow the strategies below to turn your *Junk-Food Junkie* around. To learn more about sugar and how to reverse your *Junk-Food Junkie's* intake, check out my book *Beat Sugar Addiction Now! for Kids*.

Strategies for the *Junk-Food Junkie*

With a *Junk-Food Junkie*, you are dealing with an addict—or close to it. Your child can no more regulate her intake of junk food than most adults can. Keeping junk food out of the house, eating healthy snacks between meals, serving appropriate portions, and limiting treats to one a day are essential techniques that can help you manage your *Junk-Food Junkie*.

If you have a sweet tooth, then you know how difficult it can be to resist the urge to indulge in cookies, candy, or cake when these foods are in your house. For your *Junk-Food Junkie*, it will be next to impossible to resist, which is why it is necessary to keep no more than one junk treat in the house at a time. A good tip, and one that will give your child a sense of control, is to take your *Junk-Food Junkie* shopping each week to pick his treat for the week.

This weekly treat will serve as an enticement that you need to turn your *Junk-Food Junkie* around. "You can have your cookies after you finish your meal" or "Eat your fruit first and then you can have a treat for a snack" are two examples of eat-then-treat. If your child screams for more than one treat in the store or at home, take away her daily one-treat privilege until she can behave.

Allow your *Junk-Food Junkie* ample time and space to act out if she feels crummy. Other techniques for helping your child cope are having her get exercise, go outside, and drink plenty of water.

Your child needs to learn why it is so important to limit added sugar, salt, and solid fats in his diet and that he must eat the good, healthy stuff first before the junk. Start by teaching your child which foods and beverages are in the junk category and which are in the healthy food category. Your *Junk-Food Junkie* will most likely have a predisposition to turn to junk food when he gets stressed and will most likely always have a sweet tooth, especially if he has a relative with an addictive personality. Your goal is to teach your child that even though he has this propensity, he must always choose his food consciously and not let his taste buds lead the way.

Provide healthy snacks, especially while you are limiting the amount of junk food in your child's diet. The healthy snacks should give your child the protein and whole grains that she needs to keep her blood sugar level under control. The worst scenario for the *Junk-Food Junkie* is being superhungry. If your child gets to the point where she is screaming for a fix (candy, cookies, chips), you will be hard-pressed to calm her down enough to eat a healthy alternative.

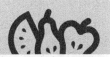

SUMMARY OF STRATEGIES FOR THE *JUNK-FOOD JUNKIE*

- Teach your *Junk-Food Junkie* which foods are considered junk and why eating too much of them is unhealthy.

- Allow your child to pick out her treat for the week.

- Limit treats to one a day, after healthy food is eaten.

- Slowly reduce the *Junk-Food Junkie*'s intake of sugar.

- Allow for a detox period.

- Being superhungry is not a good state for the *Junk-Food Junkie*; provide healthy snacks between meals.

The *Drinker*

Temperament: Slow to adapt, usually active, probably sensitive, possibly persistent

Overview: Prefers drinking calories to eating them

Diet quality: A very limited diet; low in fruits, vegetables, fiber, and grains

Christopher walks around with his bottle all day long and doesn't seem to be interested in eating food at mealtime. When he reaches three years old he prefers to drink milk at mealtimes and has little room left for dinner. Fast-forward ten years, and Christopher is drinking three cans of soda a day and eating little at mealtimes.

Drinkers prefer to get their calories from beverages than from food. This habit starts early, and it is one that needs to be remedied before it gets out of control. Baby or toddler *Drinkers* are often found walking around with the bottle or sippy cup in hand, full of milk or juice most of the day. Tween/teen *Drinkers* down two to three sodas a day and train their taste buds to prefer sweet-tasting foods, which usually translates to nutrient-deficient junk food. By the time *Drinkers* sit down for a meal, which is often a struggle, they are not hungry because of all the liquid calories that they consumed beforehand.

Some *Drinkers* seem more vulnerable than their peers, especially when they are young. They turn to the bottle for comfort and use it to self-soothe as other children would their thumb or blanket. As such, this behavior sneaks up on parents. Before they know it, their baby or toddler will not give up their bottle or sippy cup and becomes very agitated and upset when they are without it. It seems easier to give in than to fight it. What was once a cute and life-sustaining behavior has turned into a habit that is tough to break.

This vulnerability may be a sign of a sensitivity issue. It is likely that many *Drinkers* currently have or have had a hard time with the texture or taste of food. From a *Drinker*'s perspective, beverages are safe and predictable: They have a thin consistency, no texture, and are usually served at the same temperature. The taste from one bottle to the next or one glass to the next is usually identical, so there is no chance for surprises. Have your child evaluated for a sensitivity disorder if you suspect that this may be the case.

When babies are mature enough to begin eating solid foods, they are given varieties that are smooth and ground up into a thick liquid consistency. As they age, they are exposed to more textures: crunchy, tough, brittle, hard, spongy, and so on. Feeding children food with varying tastes and textures is essential as their tongue and taste buds learn to like the different tastes and textures that they are exposed to. Kids do not come into the world with too many strong likes and dislikes; rather it is mostly the foods that they are exposed to at an early age that sets their food preferences for life. The habit of drinking calories and excluding or limiting calories from solid food is the definition of a restricted, picky eater.

Strategies for the *Drinker*

There are several issues to address with the *Drinker* and thus different strategies for each:

1 Your *Drinker* drinks too many beverages before mealtime and comes to the table full. If this is the issue with your child, then limit all beverages except water within an hour of mealtime. Once your *Drinker* finishes her meal, serve your child her milk. For older children, set limits on the amount of unhealthy drinks that they are allowed per day. The average teenage boy drinks about 30 ounces of soda a day and the average teenage girl almost 20 ounces a day. Soda and other sugar-sweetened beverages not only add unnecessary calories and sugar to your child's diet, they often replace the milk and solid food that they need to consume daily to build healthy bodies and strong bones.

Do not allow your older child access to soda in your house, and teach him the importance of limiting unhealthy beverages in his diet. Explain to him that soda is a treat and should be limited to once a week. If your teen still comes to the table full, excuse him with the warning that the next time he is hungry, he can reheat his dinner. There will be no snacks, desserts, or sweetened beverages until that occurs.

2 Your *Drinker* consumes too many beverages during her meal and has little room left for food. The best strategy to break the drinking habit is to separate beverages from mealtimes. You don't need to offer a lot to drink at a meal as long as your child has had enough to drink between meals—water and milk, specifically. As long as your child is properly hydrated when she comes to the table, there is no reason to offer more than 4 to 8 ounces (120 to 235 ml) of water to help food go down smoothly.

Establish ground rules, such as *no beverages with the exception of water* until your *Drinker* eats her dinner. Even an eighteen- to twenty-four-month-old can get that concept. An older child may complain and whine at first, exclaiming that he is dying of thirst. Offer water in this situation only. Once he has eaten what is required, then it is perfectly fine to give him a glass of milk. You can return to offering milk at meals once the habit is broken, but keep an eye on it to make sure it doesn't return.

Another great strategy is to use the beverage as an incentive to get your *Drinker* to eat her meal. Implement the eat-then-treat rule often but instead of "Eat your dinner to get your treat," use the beverage as the incentive: "Once you eat your dinner, you can have your milk."

Toward a Healthy Future

Give yourself a huge pat on the back! Tackling an issue as large as picky eating is a major feat, which is why many parents let unhealthy eating habits go on way too long. You didn't because something in you knew that the way your children were eating was not good for their health.

You have learned that you need to teach your children how to eat a healthy diet and not to leave it up to their desires, wishes, and taste buds. You are now equipped with tools and strategies to work with your picky eaters so that you can turn their unhealthy eating habit around before it affects their health or potential to live a long, happy, and productive life.

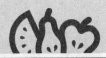

SUMMARY OF STRATEGIES FOR THE *DRINKER*

- Do not allow drinks except water within an hour of mealtime.

- Separate beverages (except water) from meals, so the *Drinker* focuses on eating, not drinking, his or her meal.

- Serve your child enough calcium-rich sources such as milk between and after meals instead.

- Use the beverage as the incentive to get your *Drinker* to eat food at mealtime.

Food and Table Rules to Live By

Have your children color in this sheet and then post it where your family usually eats.

Food and Table Rules to Live By

The 6 Food Rules

1. Eat then treat: Eat the healthy food first before having a treat.

2. One-bite rule: Everyone has to try one bite of a new food.

3. Eat a fruit or veggie with every meal and snack.

4. Limit food waste.

5. Only one dinner is served.

6. No "yuck" is allowed at the table.

The 4 Table Rules

1. Everyone has a job to do at mealtime.

2. Eat at the table only.

3. Electronics are not allowed at the table during mealtime.

4. Whoever raises his or her voice leaves the table.

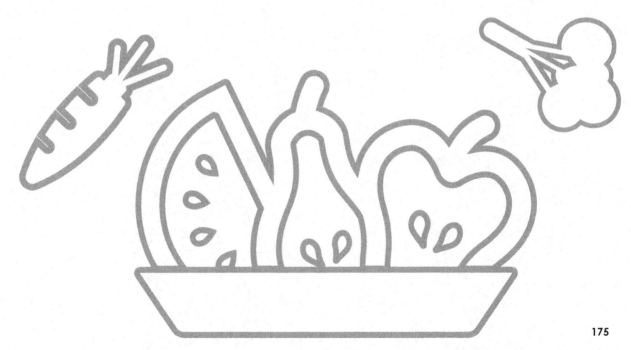

APPENDIX B

Daily Serving Guide
for Children

Daily Serving Guide for Children

Food Group	Children 2 to 3	Children 4 to 8	Boys 9 to 13	Boys 14 to 18	Girls 9 to 13	Girls 14 to 18
Total grains In ounce equivalents (oz eq)	3 oz eq	5 oz eq	6 oz eq	8 oz eq	5 oz eq	6 oz eq
Whole grains (Eat at least half of these as whole grains)	At least 1½ of the 3 oz eq	At least 2½ of the 5 oz eq	At least 3 of the 6 oz eq	At least 4 of the 8 oz eq	At least 3 of the 5 oz eq	At least 3 of the 6 oz eq
Vegetables	1 cup	1½ cups	2½ cups	3 cups	2 cups	2½ cups
Fruit	1 cup	1½ cups	1½ cups	2 cups	1½ cups	1½ cups
Milk	2 cups	2½ cups	3 cups	3 cups	3 cups	3 cups
Protein foods In ounce equivalents (oz eq)	2 oz eq	4 oz eq	5 oz eq	6½ oz eq	5 oz eq	5 oz eq
Oils	3 teaspoons	4 teaspoons	5 teaspoons	6 teaspoons	5 teaspoons	5 teaspoons
Empty calories*	135 out of 1,000 calories	120 out of 1,200 to 1,400 calories	160 out of 1,800 calories	265 out of 2,200 calories	120 out of 1,600 calories	160 out of 1,800 calories
Added sugar calories**	67 calories	60 calories	80 calories	132 calories	60 calories	80 calories

These recommendations are based on children getting less than thirty minutes per day of moderate physical activity. Your children may need more or less depending on their activity level or any other special circumstances.

Source: www.choosemyplate.gov, accessed February 2013

*Discretionary calories are the calories remaining after your child has consumed the recommended food and beverages from the food groups listed above.

**The American Heart Association recommends that only half of the empty calories come from added sugar.

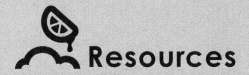 # Resources

Websites

www.buildhealthykids.com
Build Healthy Kids is a program developed for the busy family. Parents learn to focus on making one change a month as a family based on nutritional guidelines, with the information and support provided by Dr. Deb.

www.choosemyplate.gov
Choosemyplate.gov provides the information you need to make healthful changes. Go to www.choosemyplate.gov/supertracker-tools/daily-food-plans.html to create a personal daily food plan.

Books

Beat Sugar Addiction Now! for Kids: The Cutting-Edge Program That Gets Kids Off Sugar Safely, Easily, and Without Fights and Drama. By Jacob Teitelbaum, M.D., and Deborah Kennedy, Ph.D. (Fair Winds Press, 2012)

Raising a Sensory Smart Child: The Definitive Handbook for Helping Your Child with Sensory Processing Issues by Lindsey Biel and Nancy Peske (Penguin Books: Revised edition, 2009)

Acknowledgments

I thank my family for giving me the time, support, and freedom to pursue my love of writing and to share my love of food with the world. My husband provides the steady foundation from which I can fly; thank you Michael. I also count my blessings for having met occupational therapist Randy Fedoruk at Sensation Station, who opened my eyes to the complexity of sensory disorders.

About the Author

Deborah Kennedy, Ph.D., has studied food her entire life, learning to cook at age four, becoming a chef, and then obtaining her doctorate in nutritional biochemistry with a focus on nutrition and behavior from Tufts University. She is the coauthor of *Beat Sugar Addiction Now! for Kids* (Fair Winds Press, 2012) and the self-published *Nutrition Bites*. Known as Dr. Deb, she founded the program Build Healthy Kids, which is currently in more than 250 schools nationwide from Alaska to Maine. She sits on the board of directors of Cat Cora's not-for-profit Chefs for Humanity. Dr. Deb was the founder of the Integrative Therapies Program for Children with Cancer at Children's Hospital of New York-Presbyterian. She was the associate director of nutrition at Yale-Griffin Prevention Research Center, where she worked with David Katz, M.D., and helped to develop the algorithm that went on to create NuVal scores. She also worked with Mehmet Oz, M.D., at Columbia Presbyterian Hospital in the field of integrative medicine. She lives in Connecticut with her husband and two boys, who are the center of her life.

Index

Also Available

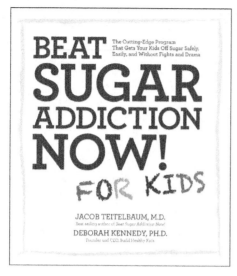

Beat Sugar Addiction Now! for Kids
978-1-59233-523-7

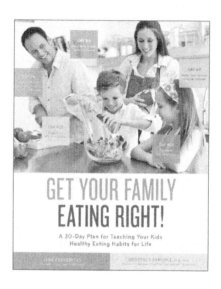

Get Your Family Eating Right
978-1-59233-550-3

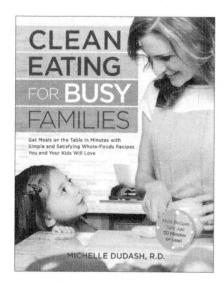

Clean Eating for Busy Families
978-1-59233-514-5

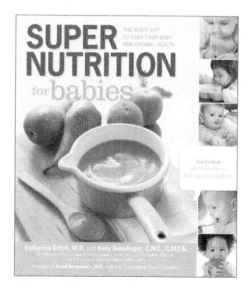

Super Nutrition for Babies
978-1-59233-503-9